AF573823

ALWAYS AND ALWAYS

ALWAYS AND ALWAYS

The Wartime Letters of Hugh and Margaret Williams

EDITED BY KATE DUNN

JOHN MURRAY
Albemarle Street, London

First published in 1995
by John Murray (Publishers) Ltd.,
50 Albemarle Street, London W1X 4BD

A catalogue record for this book is available from the British Library

ISBN 0-7195-5472-1

Typeset in Linotron Imprint by
Rowland Phototypesetting Ltd,
Bury St Edmunds, Suffolk

Printed and bound in Great Britain by
The University Press, Cambridge

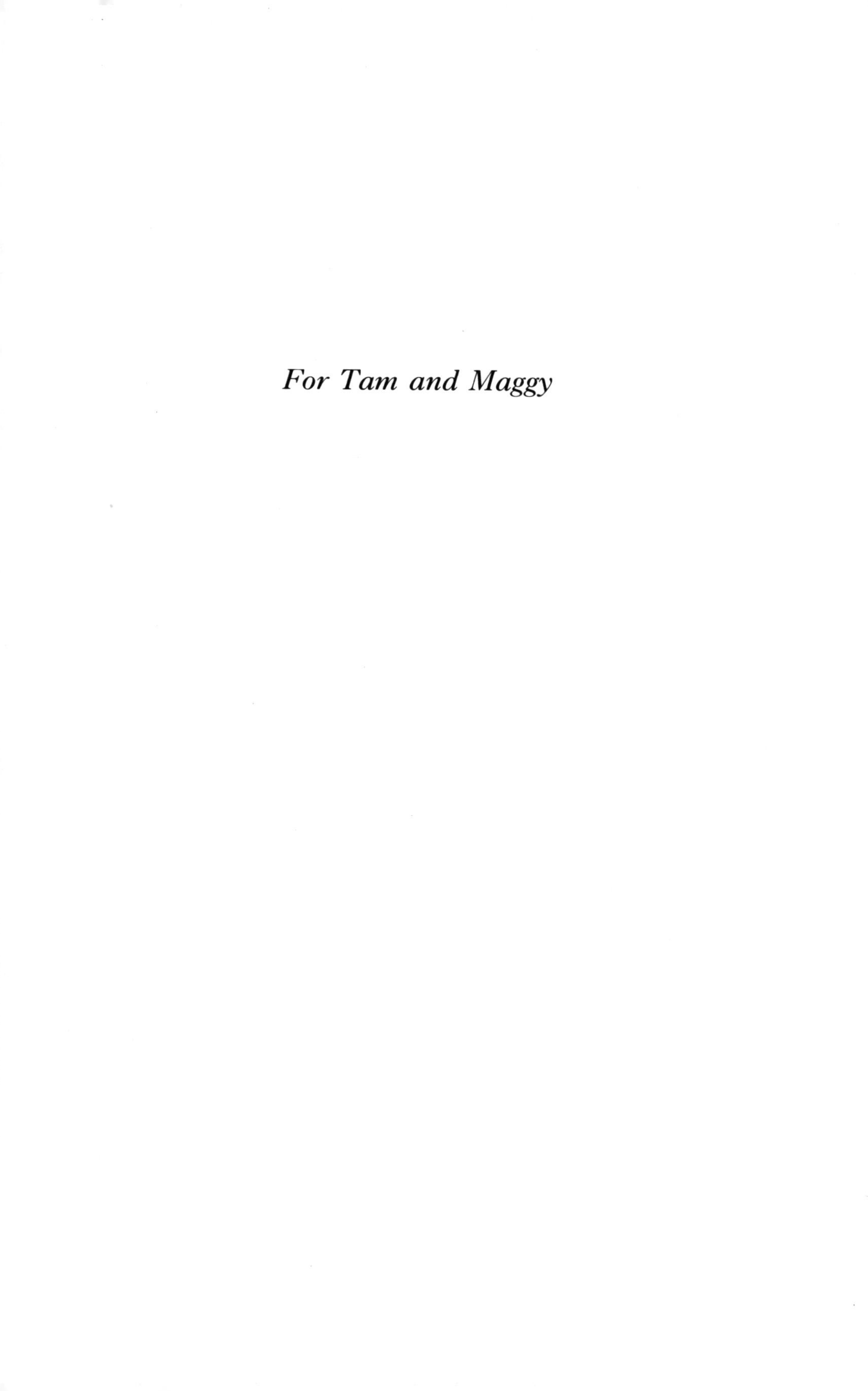

For Tam and Maggy

Contents

Illustrations

We are grateful to the following for allowing us to reproduce photographs: Simon Williams Nos. 1, 4, 6, 10, 16; Tom Dunn No. 2; Prue Dunn Nos. 3, 5, 7, 8, 11, 14, 19; Hugo Williams Nos. 9, 15, 17; Imperial War Museum No. 12; Loo Arkwright No. 13

Acknowledgements

Working on the wartime correspondence of my grandfather Tam and his second wife Margaret has been an enormous pleasure. Some of the letters were tied with pink silk ribbon, as all such letters should be, and the ones Tam received from Margaret during the North African campaign in 1943 still contained trickles of desert sand which streamed out when I first opened them. In preparing this collection I have tried to arrange the letters in chronological order; in instances where they are undated I have inserted them where they fitted best. Occasionally Tam sent Margaret poems he had written. I have included these next to the letters they accompanied.

I am grateful to my uncles Hugo and Simon Williams and my aunt Polly Havers for first allowing me to browse through the correspondence and then permitting me to publish it. They have been most helpful with background information and in providing photographs and I have been touched by their encouragement throughout the project.

I am indebted to my mother Prue and my aunt Loo for their enthusiastic endorsement of my work and their tolerance of the numerous telephone calls checking on various details. My thanks also to Barrie Hinksman for his unstinting support and to the Actor's Charitable Trust for their generous patronage.

The Trustees of the Imperial War Museum have kindly given permission for the photograph of Tam on active service to be reproduced, and I am also grateful to my father John Dunn, Nigel Seals of *The Spotlight*, Sarah Johnson, the Lady Elizabeth Clyde and Jeremy Clyde for their help with research.

Finally I would like to thank Sarah Molloy and Caroline Knox for sharing my conviction that Tam and Margaret's correspondence is unique in its power to move, amuse and inform, and for helping me to share it with a wider audience.

Introduction

Hugh Anthony Glanmôr Williams was born on 6 March 1904. He became known as Tam because when his Welsh mother Silver was pregnant with him, she referred to her bump as her 'Tamèd' or 'Little Bit'. Tam's father died of tuberculosis in 1905 and Silver remarried when her son was seven to Alexander Mordaunt Shairp (known as Sandy), a successful playwright.

His step-father's creative influence helped to steer Tam towards a career in the theatre. In 1921 he went to the Royal Academy of Dramatic Art where he met and fell in love with a fellow student, Gwynne Whitby. After a tempestuous four-year engagement that was repeatedly broken off, the couple were married in 1925. The relationship was dealt a serious blow the following year when the notorious American star Tallulah Bankhead saw Tam play Bertie Lennox in *The Best People*[1] at the Lyric Theatre in London. Without actually saying that she required him to be stripped, washed and brought to her tent, she made it clear that she wanted the beautiful young man to be in her next play. In the December of that year Tam and Talullah opened in *The Gold Diggers*[2] and from then on his marriage to Gwynne was seriously under threat. In a bid to save the day, Silver and Sandy contacted the producer Dion Boucicault and arranged for the troubled young couple to be whisked out of harm's way to Australia. They were away for eighteen months appearing in a repertoire of five plays. Margaret's first glimpse of Tam was when he appeared on stage in Sydney during this tour. She was immediately smitten. When he and Gwynne returned to England the *status quo* had been restored, and in spite

1. *The Best People* by David Grey and Avery Hopwood opened on 16 March 1926 at the Lyric Theatre and ran for 308 performances.
2. *The Gold Diggers* by Avery Hopwood opened on 14 December 1926 at the Lyric Theatre and ran for 179 performances.

of further infidelities, in 1931 she gave birth to their first child, a daughter, christened Penelope but known, in a compromise, as Loo since Tam had wished her to be called Llewella. At the end of the following year a second daughter, Prudence, was born. The arrival of the girls failed to provide the necessary cement for the marriage and in 1933 Tam and Gwynne agreed to separate.

By now Tam's acting career was flourishing. In the next four years he appeared in seven plays in both London and New York, scoring a personal success in an early study in homosexuality, *The Green Bay Tree*, written by his step-father. During this time he made twenty-one films, amongst them *Rome Express*, *Bitter Sweet* and most famously David Lean's *David Copperfield* with Freddie Bartholomew and W.C. Fields. However, Tam's life was changed irrevocably in the December of 1937, for it was then that he fell in love with Margaret Vyner.

Margaret cultivated a certain vagueness about the year of her birth but it was probably 1914, on the 3rd of December. Most of her early life was lived in Armidale, New South Wales. Her grandfather was Sir Richard Vyner, Baronet, reputedly descended from the Richard Vyner who made the coronation regalia for the restoration of Charles II. He made his living laying out English gardens in Australia and disappearing before they too disappeared in the summer drought. Her father Robert was educated at Birkenhead School in England before returning home to Australia to set up a sheep station. He married Ruby Nicholson, a great beauty, and Margaret Leila was their only child. Robert seems to have been quite a character, dousing his car with petrol when it broke down and setting light to it, leaving his wife and daughter in the shade of a coolabar tree until somone noticed the smoke and came to rescue them. His marriage to Ruby was not happy and he eventually ran off with a hairdresser named Irma. Margaret had the best available education at Frensham School in New South Wales, and thereafter went to an eccentric finishing school called Cherry's. At the age of nineteen she booked her passage to Southampton, but having borrowed £100 from a doctor she met on board, she jumped ship at Naples. With the loan and a refund she secured for missing the last week of the voyage, she travelled overland to Paris. Here she headed straight for the Rue St Florentine and the salon of Jean Patou. Meltingly beautiful, the great French couturier hired Margaret to work as a model the moment he saw her. During this time she holidayed at the fashionable resort of Le Touquet. One evening in a nightclub she caught sight of the Welsh actor who had so impressed her five years before in Australia. She managed to secure an introduction to him, but later Tam denied all recollection of this meeting. Shortly afterwards Margaret left Paris to try her luck in London. In 1935 she was at the height of her powers: Cole Porter mythologized her loveliness in his famous song 'You're the Top' from the musical *Anything Goes*: 'You're the top, you're an ocean liner / You're the top, you're Margaret Vyner.' It was not surprising that Norman Hartnell, dress designer to the new young Queen Elizabeth, welcomed Margaret as Patou had done, nicknaming her 'Bunch of Flowers'. For some months she was an adornment to the London social scene.

In the closing weeks of 1937 she heard that Hugh Williams was shortly to leave for New York, to appear in a comedy called *Once is Enough* by Frederick Lonsdale. Seeing her chance Margaret auditioned for the part of the soubrette and was asked to join the company. They sailed for New York in December on the SS *Washington* and one evening Tam sent a note to her table asking her to join him for a glass of champagne. Margaret declined, saying she preferred to drink milk, but this time there was undoubtedly a *coup de foudre* between them. When they docked they were welcomed by the play's producers wearing dinner jackets who whisked then straight to a party and Tam was able to persuade Margaret to book into the hotel where he was staying, the Gotham on Fifth Avenue. After laying siege to her for eight days, on 8 January 1938 they became lovers, an anniversary that both of them marked fervently in later years. In one of his earliest letters to her, a note sent up to her room in the hotel, Tam writes,

> You're sweet and I love you and you're the prettiest girl in New York and you scratch my head so beautifully and you make such wonderful love and I like you and you're such a baby and you're kind and you live upstairs and you wear pretty clothes and for those reasons and many more, I invite you to dine with me.

Both their careers continued to move apace. In 1938 Tam made one West End appearance and four films, while Margaret appeared in three movies herself. In spite of these diversions their feelings for each other continued to grow and before long Tam was sending urgent little notes to this effect:

> I hate Tam.
> But I love Margaret.
> Please oh Please send me a telegram saying you love me and promising to marry me and make me nicer.

I hope you're better today my pretty.
Do we dine?
My love to you.

Tam was back in Hollywood in 1939 where he made three more films, including the classic version of *Wuthering Heights* in which he played Hindley to Laurence Olivier's Heathcliffe. In spite of the burgeoning of his career, the threat of war in Europe was so imminent that he felt obliged to enlist, although at thirty-five he was well above the required age limit. In April 1939 he joined the Territorial Army, signing up as a private in the Queen's Westminsters. On 1 September he was called up into the regular army and two days later Britain declared war on Germany.

For the first six months of the war Tam served as a soldier, an experience that he hated, as the following letter to Margaret shows.

Darling,

This is utterly unreal and quite quite awful. I didn't know it could be so awful. I feel trapped and afraid and resentful and very miserable. Tomorrow I shall be in London for the afternoon to see you. It's only a few hours.

My love my darling, Tam.

However, life improved for him when on 9 March 1940 he received his commission into the 8th Battalion of the Devonshire Regiment. Three months later he and Margaret were married. In his letter to her mother asking her permission for the match, he describes himself and his life in this way:

Since the war my income has become a decimal point and my poor wretched family – my mother, my wife and two daughters – are suffering wretchedly as a result. No one can say what will happen after the war but basing my income on the last seven or eight years I shall be able to support both them and Margaret very comfortably. I was divorced last year, but my wife and I hadn't lived together for more than five years before I met Margaret so that she is in no way responsible. What else is there to tell you? I'm thirty six, like Margaret an only child, I'm not a very good soldier but I was quite a good actor, I'm not very fond of animals, I prefer babies. I'm punctual, superstitious, careless, inclined to worry, healthy, not wise, but very loving towards your daughter and my own personal Peace Aims are to make her happy, take care of her, and give her the kind of life that will keep her interested, amused and contented.

The wedding took place at St Ethelburga's Church in Bishopsgate on 21 June 1940. For the next eighteen months Tam's military career consisted of highlights such as guarding Staines Bridge and defending the south coast at Bexhill-on-Sea. Margaret did her war work too, serving lunches at the British Restaurant in the Strand.

In the middle of 1941 the film director Michael Powell asked if Tam might be released from the army to assist the war effort by making a series of morale-boosting films. There followed a year of marital bliss for him and Margaret. She became pregnant with their son Hugo (the poet Hugo Williams) and he starred in films such as *Ships With Wings*, *Secret Mission*, *One of Our Aircraft is Missing*, and *The Day will Dawn*.

The end of 1942 saw Tam back in the army. Using the influence of his friend Major John Hannay (Johnny), he was attached to Phantom. This was a secret intelligence regiment whose brief was to locate the Allied forward positions and act as a direct communication link between the forward patrols and command headquarters. Phantom informed the British, Americans and Canadians what their forward troops were doing and how the enemy was responding. Units were at Dieppe with the Commandoes, in France with the SAS, at Arnhem with the First Airborne Division and in Germany until the surrender. It had the character of a colourful private army and contained many who were to be become famous in later years, including two Privy Councillors, three life peers, the master of a Cambridge College, three professors, a film star, a sculptor, a Law Lord, a leader writer, an ambassador, a steward of the Jockey Club, a Commissioner of the Metropolitan Police and several authors.

As well as Johnny, Tam became friends with Major J.A. Warre MC (Tony), Captain S.S. Demetriadi (Dick Springett) and Lieutenant Lord Charles Banbury (The Bag). Margaret in her turn had the support of her great friend Jasmine Bligh, and also Charles and Vi Eaton and Tommy and Eliza Clyde, who were neighbours in the village of Dorney near Windsor.

These then, are the cast of characters in the correspondence which follows. The letters themselves are full of observation and detail of the daily lives of people both at home and at the Front: tiny personal scraps of information, footnotes to the great historical events that were occurring all around them.

In his kit Tam always carried a poem written by his father to

Silver when he was dying. He and Margaret used to quote from it when times were hard, as they frequently were during the war years.

> Troubles I have full many great and small,
> And ever am by sickness sore oppress'd
> Yet, thank the gods! The sweets out taste the gall,
> For I am loved and love – what boots the rest?

Above all, these are love letters and this emotion burns through in all its manifestations, from the first flush of passion to jealousy and even disenchantment. Like millions of other couples who lived through the desperate months of the Blitz, through reversals such as Dunkirk and Arnhem, the triumphs of the North African campaign, the long periods of separation and the months, indeed years, of waiting and longing for the war to end, Tam and Margaret had to come to terms with the unrealistic expectations of each other that the war engendered. It was an incalculable strain and this is painfully evident in some of their correspondence: Tam's possessiveness and feelings of insecurity and the questions surrounding Margaret's fidelity are among the issues they confronted and bravely attempted to resolve. What appears to have sustained them, and possibly countless other couples in the same situation, was the need to love and be loved in a world that appeared to be disintegrating all around them. What boots the rest?

The Letters

1939–42

Before the British Public
I was once a leading man,
Now behind a British Private
I just follow if I can.

Margaret to Tam London, (undated) 1939

My own, my very own darling,

Have just been up to our room and was about to go to bed, but when I thought of getting into bed alone, without you, I very nearly rushed to the station to follow you. So finding myself in this very loving sentimental frame of mind, I thought it best to come downstairs again and write my love and longing to you.

Oh my darling you have been the most tender, loving, thoughtful, thrilling and amusing lover to me this weekend. And in spite of the passion we have and always show each other, when we are alone it is the tenderness of lying asleep beside you and waking to find you there again which I miss the most of all.

This relationship (I use this bad word for want of a better) which we have must be cherished for surely it is one of the most perfect to have existed. I love you so my Blackie,[1] belong to me always as I shall to you.

Forgive this passionate dissertation my darling, but my heart is very full as it always is when we have to leave each other.

Until the 26th darling,
Your very own M.

1. Blackie was Margaret's nickname for Tam, perhaps because when they met he had thick, coal-black hair.

Margaret to Tam London, 16 October 1939

My beloved,

You are being so really wonderful and cheerful about everything and I know how really wretched and miserable you must be down there.[1] Particularly now that the others have gone. However I console myself by thinking that as they have a very particular and special job for you, they had to make the others officers first to sort of get them settled. Then in a few days time they will come to you and say 'Tamèd, we have come to dress and bathe you and escort you to your new quarters – if you are ready, of course.'

Tell me about the rabbits!!

I adore you above and beyond all else,
Always and always, your M.

1. Training in Aldershot.

Margaret to Tam London, 16 October 1939

Oh my own darling,

What absolute dejection and utter misery it is here without you. I love you so much and miss you so much that at the moment I feel quite suicidal and can't imagine how I shall go on without you.

Bitch bugger shit. I loathe this bloody war and all it is doing to us. However, we *must* both try not to let our eyes waver for a single moment from the very top of the heavenly moments which I know are waiting way over there. I can get by with my chin up if you can. I can be strong and I *will* be strong because of our love for each other. I'd die without you darling, of this be sure.

It was such heaven having you here for those few days and already I feel I *must* see you again terribly soon. I do hope you are comfortable where you are darling. Take care of your arm and keep it clean and leave the scabs on as long as possible, otherwise the scars will be horrible.[1]

Oh my beloved, just love me and come to me as often as you can. I long to see you and be with you always,

For always and always, your own M.

1. Tam was suffering from an outbreak of impetigo.

Margaret to Tam London, 8 November 1939

Darlingest One,

So sorry to have missed you when you rang this evening. I did ring back but you were not there, and a very nice man told me you were going on night operations at 9. What absolute hell and the ground will be so wet. I do hope they don't make you lie down darling. Take care of your cold *please*. You must have had a hell of a day too. How I hate to think of you doing anything but the most wonderful, exciting and elegant things. Oh dear! As usual when you have been with me for a day or two, I'm plunged into the depths of loneliness, misery and despair when you go back. We did have a lovely two days and at least now we have something to look forward to – next time. I pray it will be soon.

Today I did odd bits and pieces but nothing special – Oh, no money for the 'Queen' thing – *they* are writing about me. HELL.

God bless and take care of you my beloved,

Always and always, your M.

Tam to Margaret Aldershot, November 1939

My Darling,

Life has descended with a boomps-a-daisy from the elysian heights of Saturday and Sunday – we arrived back to find I was Platoon Commander for the week – naturally I haven't the faintest idea of what to do and I want at least three weeks rehearsal and a week on the road. However, I've had a bit of luck for practically everyone is sick – two inoculations yesterday – a prod and a scowl in the right arm from one gentleman for Tetanus and a prick and a chuckle from another in the left for Typhoid – it's made me very stiff from the waist up – so disappointing – but thank God I'm not as bad as most of them.

Saw the Colonel yesterday about regiments and went bang for the Welsh Guards and this morning my Company Commander sent for me and said he'd write to the Commander of one of the battalions, which is excellent, for if he'd waited he might have found out what a cunt I am.

Goodnight my pretty, longing for Saturday, forgive the most dreary letter – my mind is full of maps and compass bearings and drill movements and Military Law and the Theory of Small Arms Fire and my body full of lock jaw and typhoid, but I adore you – you must be beginning to know that.

Forever and ever,

Tamèd

P.S. More rumours this morning – the favourite's Folkestone – I've started one that the whole battalion is moving to the Piccadilly at two for one.

Margaret to Tam London, 15 November 1939

Tamèd my beloved,

Oh my angel heart what a wonderful and exciting two days we have had. One might almost hope that our luck has changed. Nevertheless, as I said at dinner on Sunday, in spite of all the sadness and disappointments we've had during the last two years I still think I did right in staying on that boat, you and me together love, never mind the weather love. Thinking of you and loving you always,

Your M.

Margaret to Tam London, 21 November 1939

My beloved darling,

Have just put the telephone away having just spoken to you at the Green Room.[1] I told you I loved you. Well, that was not quite true – if there is such a word, I Love You^4 (you remember algebra?). I adore you, you are so very dear and precious darling. And when we have to part each time in order that you may go away to some town or place I've never heard of and do a lot of things I can't imagine, it leaves me lonely, puzzled and unhappy. For although I've heard war talk since the day I was born, talk of the last and possibility of another, I've never been able to completely understand the reasons for it. It seems that we, the middle and lower classes, fight for the lost ambitions and ideals of those who are already in, or have fought mentally to be in, the upper strata. This thing called war has absolutely nothing to do with us or our friends and contemporaries. It's my story of you cleaning other people's 'lavs' all over again. What rot I talk darling. I'm chatting again I fear me. Or am I? The fact remains and will always and always, I love you darling mine,

Your very own,

Thine M.

1. Tam belonged to the Green Room, a London club for actors, now situated in Adam Street off the Strand.

Tam to Margaret Letter by hand, November 1939

Oh my dear, my darling Margaret,

Will you please *please* lend me £1 – I want to buy some flowers for somebody – it's her birthday and I love her so and I think she'd be disappointed if I didn't give her just something – if I were rich I'd build her a house somewhere they have palm trees. I love her, I love her.

Tam to Margaret Aldershot, 23 November 1939

My Darling,

Thank you for your letter this morning and my beautiful vest, pants and torch. You're a wonderful woman with an apparently inexhaustible supply of money to buy my little comforts – can it be that you're feathering my nest?

Very weary tonight – digging weapons' pits and P.T. – How's your cold my darling? Please get it well – I love you. I love you and more than I want peace on earth and goodwill towards men, I want you to go on being idiotic enough to love me.

For ever, for ever and always and a day I shall be yours my Margaret,
Tam

Margaret to Tam 28 November 1939

My beloved darling,

Have just come home having had quite a good day, for it looks as if I *might* get a job in a new show starring Bebe Daniels and Ben Lyon[1] and a lot of others, but will know more towards the end of the week. However, it is nice to even be a 'perhaps'.

Darling what a heavenly weekend we had, it will be a time to be remembered, don't you agree?

I'm being good and faithful and loving you darling and will be
Always and always your M.

1. Bebe Daniels and Ben Lyon were an American acting couple. They specialized in light comedy and musicals and in December 1940 opened in *Hee Haw* at the London Palladium, without Margaret, as it transpired.

Margaret to Tam London, 4 December 1939

My very own beloved,

Many many thanks my darling for a lovely birthday. No, don't smile, we both knew that presents are impossible now but as I told you before my love, you are my present always. And as long as you are towards me as you were these last two days, 'What boots the rest?' You've got all the things in you that I want and desire passionately and tenderly. We'll be able to give each other all the presents we wish to later on. The house with the palm trees I accept with pleasure and gratitude. I shall move in on January 8th 1942. I'm posting your sponge bag to you by the same post as this little letter,

I love you and I miss you always, M.

Margaret to Tam London, 7 December 1939

My beloved,

I am in bed and it is now only about 11pm. Except for last night when we went to the Café de Paris and were home at 1pm I have been in bed at about this time. Good girl?

I absolutely adore you, you angel beloved darling sweetheart, but I can not obey you and go away, for I have *absolutely* no money and am therefore rooted to the spot. It breaks my heart for I do so want to buy you the things you want on account of I love you and I'm your own M always.

Tam to Margaret Aldershot, 13 December 1939

OH! My Dear Girl! Have a look at these – what are we to do? Hilarious.

'Is it just war time emotionalism? Are you marrying the man or his uniform? Do you really know each other well enough?'

'When you go out together would he dance more with you – his wife – than with other women?'

'Is he equally popular with men and women? . . .'

'Will he ever say in a loud, cold voice, 'You'd better not have another drink? . . .'

'Have you ever seen him in mufti? . . . (Has he adapted himself well to his war life, or is he a grouser?)'

'Would he be a good companion at breakfast and on Monday mornings? . . .'

'Do you agree on money questions? . . . (Whether a wife should have a definite allowance or whether the husband should dole out money when she asks for it)'

'Is he sensible about money?'

'Have you spent a certain amount of time in each other's home? . . . (Would it not be possible to spend at least a weekend with each other's family? You see people in a much truer light when they are at home.)'.

Tam to Margaret Aldershot, Friday 16 December 1939
Military Transport Lecture

Oh my dear Girl,

I've never been so cold in all my life – the only time I get warm is when I'm sitting under the infra red lamp at the hospital and then I'm so frightened of the massage to follow that I still shiver. The masseuse is the littlest woman you ever saw but with a twist of her pretty fingers she has me quite literally under her thumb – not only under her thumb but bouncing off my chair and onto the floor.

Thank you for all the jobs you did for me this week – you're a wonderful woman and how clever I am to have found you. I fear this is a somewhat disjointed letter – but I have to look up every now and then to pretend I'm listening – it's all about petrol and carburetters which I cannot understand and refuse to recognise as being of any military value.

Saw Robert Donat in 'Mr Chips'[1] last night – what a really magnificent performance – so simple, so untheatrical, so beautifully thought out and superbly executed and for a young man quite excellent I thought. A lovely picture and I sobbed noisily and not so prettily as my daughter Penelope.[2]

I love you so much my dear and lovely Margaret and the only other thing I miss half as much as not seeing you is the sun – if I can have you and the sun after the war I shall count myself a King.
My love to you forever,
Tam

P.S. Johnny[3] is trying to decode the cypher on my lighter.

1. Robert Donat (1905–58), actor, starred in numerous films including *Goodbye Mr Chips*.
2. Penelope was Tam's elder daughter by his first marriage to the actress Gwynne Whitby. Known as Loo, she was born in 1931.
3. Major J. M. Hannay, a friend of Tam's who adored Margaret. After the war he worked as a director of the Savoy Hotel. He died in 1972.

1940–2

Tam to Margaret Bexhill-on-Sea, 3 January 1940

My dear, my darling Margaret,

I want to be with you and live somewhere warm with you and if this bloody war is going to go lingering on then I'm going to get terribly impatient – for I really have no interest in life unless it is to be with you nearly *all* the time. Something quite horrible happened this Christmas and I'm distressed and considerably disturbed about it. It has entered my head – and now I cannot remove the doubt – that I'm not nearly good enough for you. I admit it's preposterous and ridiculous, but there it is and it's most annoying so be nice my darling and write and explain that I'm quite wrong.

I'm Company Orderly Sergeant tomorrow – a bloody job. Keep warm – and keep happy. Even though I'm not good enough for you I *do* love you so badly. So very very badly, I always will – always – for ever – and ever.

Tam

Margaret to Tam Chelsea, 18 January 1940

Oh my darling,

What absolute bliss it is to feel a little better, even if I am bright yellow. The old doc says I'm to stay here until all the yellow has gone. Absolute hell. Silver[1] rang up and said she would come to see me today or tomorrow, and that Loo went back looking as pretty as a picture. Bless her.

Mollie Sullivan[2] wants me to be a bridesmaid in March. Methinks I'd feel rather an old bag and a bit of a fraud into the bargain. I've a feeling that one is supposed to be a virgin and never to have had jaundice, but I'm not sure.

It is just wonderful to know that you are feeling a bit better darling. I hate to think of you working your way through a maze of catarrh (can't spell the horrid thing) while I lie here being peacefully administered to by pretty women.

Oh I give up.

My beloved black one, always thy M.

1. Tam's mother.
2. Mollie Heineman, née Sullivan.

Tam to Margaret Bexhill-on-Sea, 7 March 1940

You were very sweet just now on the telephone – a pity for now I feel worse, if you'd been beastly I'd have said, 'Nuts, why shouldn't I behave like a shit anyway?'

I love you very much and I'm distressed as deep as I love you and rather frightened too. If I lose you then – then – I don't know really but I wouldn't be happy ever again. Don't keep this letter – tear it up or burn it or send it to *The Times* – but don't forget what it says.

My love to you my very valuable one,
Tam

Margaret to Tam Chelsea, (undated) 1940

My own Precious One,

Now let me see, I'm sure I had something to tell you first of all. Oh yes, of course. I adore you. Oh my darling, what a long time it seems since I last saw you. So hurry on, Saturday. I'm longing to see you and I'm hating doing all this packing up without you. You are such a help when packing!!! I love you. Had dinner and was in bed about 11.30 last night – good girl. Found your darling letter on the tray when I woke up. Now about you're not being good enough for me, let's do away with that thought immediately, on account of I think you are absolute perfection, even when ill, and all I want is for this ridiculous war to end and everyone to leave us alone to love and enjoy each other.

Oh my darling, just go on loving me and believing in me and I'll never let you down in anything that matters. All I refuse to do is insult the same people as you – I must choose my own victims. Always and always my beloved, thy M.

Tam to Margaret Yelverton, Devon, 29 March 1940

Margaret my darling,

A letter from you this morning to make the wind and the rain seem like a spring day. Well, Yelverton is certainly on the Moor, and the Moor seems a foreboding piece of country in the middle of Devon, and Devon is the heart of England and England is where I have no heart to be. That's rather in the vein of Viscount Castleross, but you can sing it to the tune of 'California Here We

Comc', 'Forty Second St', 'Monterey', or 'Over the Border'.It was nice of you to remember to write to Johnny – he's very cheery and keeps me from feeling too unutterably lonely, but his snoring at night is such unearthly bellowing that I purchased ear wads from Boots this morning. Last night I awoke five times thinking that he was in pain – ill – dying – coming – and lastly that I was on fire.

My journey down was pleasant, but the engine was going the wrong way and my heart was left behind at Waterloo and my tummy was turning over and over. Remember only that I love you.
Tam

Tam to Margaret Devon, Sunday 1 April 1940

Darling,

Without wishing to excite your pity unduly or bellyache extremely – will you remember that I'm not very happy and very worried and all the time frightened. It's twenty years since I was a terrified little boy at that preposterous Haileybury and it's horrible having the same kind of feeling when one's hair has turned to silver. Alright I think so far, but I'm not very good at minding my P's and Q's – I still think a P is something I have to get up for in the middle of the night and a Q is a line of people waiting to see me act.

This course we're running is going to make a rear bloody Admiral of me if it doesn't send me nuts first – but darling what I mean is – write to me please, your letters mean so much.

If by any chance you're by the stage door of His Majesty's you'll see a little shop that sells glass and cocktail things, will you send me a dropper for angastura bitters?
Your very orderly officer and rather disorderly lover,
Tam

Margaret to Tam Chelsea, 2 April 1940

My beloved Tamèd,

Oh dear, how lonely and unhappy you sound darling, and yet the bit in your letter about P's and Q's made me laugh a lot. Just be yourself when you are out to charm and soon they'll all adore you. Doing the right thing is a lot of rot, just do what you do charmingly and everyone will be on your side I know.

Oh my beloved I do so much miss you. Shall make plans for a

visit to Devon as soon as finance allows I promise you. The postcard of you drilling your men on Dartmoor[1] looked the most depressing thing I've ever seen darling, but will you introduce me to the one third from the right. He looks very like a man I knew in Australia. It is raining like bloody stink here and I hate London more than ever.

Take care of yourself my darling and remember the crooning journalist[2] who is very much in love with you,
Always your M.

1. The picture on the postcard was of sheep on Dartmoor.
2. Margaret seems to have appeared in a short season singing at the Café de Paris, '£4 per week all told and none of the dear stuff' (their name for champagne). At the same time she was doing occasional work as a gossip columnist.

Tam to Margaret — Devon, Tuesday 4 April 1940

My Darling,

A letter from you this morning – and the sun shone turning greyness into colours and I heard a lark and saw a primrose, decided khaki wasn't a spring colour, fell a little more in love and was caught in an April shower. Later in the morning I passed a Company waiting for their dinners, just before they were called to attention I caught, 'This 'ere one's the fucking film star!' It's really more than difficult – people keep on saying 'But surely we've met before – weren't you in Llandidno for your summer holiday in '37?' or 'I've seen you round Tavistock way, I'm sure I have.' I feel a new personal high in looking a fool. I think it was Dickens who wrote 'He looked as much out of his element as a dolphin in a sentry box.' That's about the bloody strength of it.

I'm Orderly Officer in waiting – waiting now while the Adjutant has his lunch. Tomorrow this bloody course begins AND I'm Orderly Officer. Forgive me darling for being so regimental, but you can't fall down a drain without talking about the sewage.
Best love my Darling – my little fellow's turned up. I adore you.
Tam

Tam to Margaret — Devon, Wednesday evening, 4 April 1940

Oh My Dear, My Dear,

Giving a forty five minute lecture tomorrow. Accustomed as I am to public speaking I'm also accustomed to knowing what the hell I'm talking about! – How I'd love Celia[1] to play opposite me in a lecture on Patrols. No. You. You're prettier.

Continual talk here of going overseas. I am terribly overseasick, but I want no old fashioned melodrama like – 'One Night Married' or 'His Regiment Leaves at Dawn'. God how I shall act after the war – I'm loosened – my emotions all so very near the surface. Write. Write, it makes me happy. My sweet I love you,
Tam

1. Celia Johnson (1908–82), actress. She played Elizabeth to Tam's Darcy in a West End production of *Pride and Prejudice* in 1936.

Tam to Margaret — Devon, Tuesday 30 April 1940

Oh My Darling,

A little jaded, faded, wilted and fatigued old subaltern I am today – miserable and missing you so much.

I thought this morning I'd touched myself up a really good job – Entertainment Officer for the whole of 45th Division – but the Colonel has squashed it, he says he wants to keep me. Pity. I slept fairly well on the train but it was pouring with rain when I arrived and has never ceased. It was heaven seeing you and having you near again and I think I fell in love a little more – each time I say goodbye it gets just that much worse. How lucky you are to be with Johnny, will you ask him to let me have the name of that stuff he put in his petrol to make it stronger, I'm supposed to find out for the Colonel's wife.

Write to me my darling and be as good as you can. God bless and thank you for being alive.
My love forever,
Tam

Margaret to Tam — London, (undated) 1940

God Bless you my darling, wrap up well and I hope you enjoy the sandwiches.

One day you'll never have to be bored, cold, poor, unhappy, or dressed in khaki ever again. But I'll always love you, remember. Hurry home as soon as you're back.
All my love, M.

Tam to Margaret Devon, Sunday 6 May 1940

My dear Girl,

Why complicate your life? You were out on Friday at 1.15 when I telephoned – I write to ask where you will be on Saturday at 10 p.m. – no reply. Once more in your favourite position with your back to the wall, you telephone me. Almost comparable to the masterly inefficiency of our own Government and Messrs. Moss Bros. with whom I placed an order for a mackintosh holder and a forage cap last Monday and for which I paid – on Friday I received a bill for a Sam Browne. Why should you take sides with Moss Bros.? Do you want to marry Moss's Brothers or me? Think it over and let me know, and if you want some flimsy excuse let me think of one, it'll be better than yours.

What a catastrophe they made of Norway.[1] The newspapers have now reached such a pitch of fiendish imbecility that the only news one can decipher from the welter of censored information is that we have been at war with Germany since last September. The *Telegraph* invented a magnificent word for the Allied Troops being routed out of Trondheim and Namsos – Re-embarkation. God Almighty! Re-embarkation – withdrawal – retirement. Why can't England be told in the only way she should be told: in English and in English the word is Defeat. It's all very depressing. How long oh Lord how long? – How appalling if they win this time and we have to play a final.

The sun is sinking which is usually my zero hour – oh the loneliness in my heart and in my head for you. If there had to be a war why must I be in love – yet I thank God I am. I'm exceedingly and abundantly grateful to God and your mother for providing me with you. Please let's be happy.

Always,
Tam

1. On 9 April 1940 Germany invaded Norway to secure valuable sources of iron ore and to establish naval bases from which to harry the British Fleet in the North Atlantic. The Battle of Norway was waged throughout April, with Hitler retaining a firm grip on the southern, most populated areas of the country.

Tam to Margaret Eastbourne, 14 May 1940

Darling,

We arrived here at crack of dawn yesterday – it's an empty school – no water, electric light, gas, telephone, food or anything –

gradually getting organised – I have a little boy's bed – five foot long. We're here to welcome the parachutists and for coastal defence – what could be pleasanter?

Eastbourne's delightful and the people more than helpful. Luckily the owner of the local knew me so I was able to get nine gallons of beer on credit. How long we shall be here God alone knows – the news is simply horrifying and personally I think Hitler is so drunk with success and power and achievement that he may attempt an invasion by sea as well as air – it's odd to think that from Eastbourne right along the coast to Margate there are still the little Martello Towers built in 1807 or so as Watch Towers for Napoleon's flat bottomed boats that never ventured an attempt. One simply trembles at the thought of the battle that's about to begin – 2000 tanks in action already and it hasn't really started. I should think there'll be half a million casualties in the next six weeks.

I'll see you soon. Write to me and tell me what Miss Thingamy at the Bank said. God bless you my pretty. I simply adore you and I always shall.

Forever,
Tam

Tam to Margaret — Eastbourne, Thursday evening, 17 May 1940

I only get out for three hours every other day and having arranged to telephone you this evening, by a great deal of wrangling I managed to get here to do so – 'Miss Vyner is out'. I've several times been AS angry, but never more. Mr Arlen, Mr Graves, Mr Charlie Free-meal no doubt – but I'll thank you to save me the price of a Kummel by giving me sufficient warning. You'd better telephone or telegram sending your apologies – not excuses.
Signed *Highly Indignant*

P.S. You bitch, you infidel, you BAG.

Margaret to Tam — London, 22 May 1940

My darling one,

Wonder how you are feeling now. Were you very cold in the train and did you get any sleep? Each time I'm with you again makes me realise how precious you are to me, how dearly I love you, and how wonderful our lives will be after the war, more and more.

Saw Con[1] this morning. I've got the contract with me tonight and she says she thinks it is not bad at all, in fact *miles* better than she expected. There is a clause for co-star billing here and feature in America for the first year, and co-star both here and America for the second year which is *good* and *important*. So shall I sign it or keep it for you to see first?

Now darling here is the bad news. I've been over our bills etc and find the situation *very* sticky, worse than I thought in fact. There is really a great deal to pay off and if we don't we are going to have writs etc right left and centre. Tell me what you think we'd better do with our new fortune. My bank is at the moment pretty stuffy about the big overdraft. Sorry about all this darling, but it must be said and it seems a shame to spend our precious hours saying it.

Oh I do hope I can see you again soon my love. I do adore you so much and long to be with you forever and always, your own M.

1. Tam's theatrical agent, Constance Chapman.

Tam to Margaret Eastbourne, 22 May 1940

Oh My Darling,

What a lovely evening to end this of sudden miseries – I've been alone all day which means I've thought – which again is the very worst thing one can do these days. I think one must be without any feeling at all, without heart, without blood in one's veins or intelligence in one's head, not to experience the most sickening, crushing, hopeless feeling of utter and unalterable futile calamity. When you calculate that in seven days over half a million people have been killed and then you think that for every single person killed four or five are left desolate and grief stricken and probably unprovided for and then think again of all the hundreds and thousands who are now homeless, without money, without their clothes, their possessions, their means of earning a living. Then think once more that it all happened just exactly the same when I was a little boy of ten. No two wars are the same, there are always new weapons, new methods of attack, but the greatest difference between the 1914–18 war and this one is not a material one – it's deeper and more dreadful. Their generation went to battle filled with honour and glory, with poets singing their songs as they rode away to die – with flags waving and bands playing – feeling like heroes crusading to save the civilised world. But what of us? We're mute and without a song on our lips or hope in our heart. . . Think again – Louvain which is now a burning shattered shambles was only properly recovered from the last war two years ago. Liège, gallant Liège of 1914 – still the last fort firing in 1940. Think of Richmond Park, of those soldiers still in hospital blue, still with wounds unhealed after twenty years – how has the world progressed since the youth of yesterday died to save it? If Mr J.B. Priestley had collaborated with God he couldn't have conceived of a more tragic experiment with time. Am I ten or thirty six? I'm sitting in what was once a classroom, as I was twenty six years ago – the Allied Armies are avoiding rout in the same Belgian villages and on the same rivers – the Meuse, the Somme – as they were twenty-six years ago – Brussels fallen – Paris in danger – just exactly the same.

Forgive me my darling – I said at the beginning it was foolish to think but it's hard not to. Somebody interrupted me there, it's now Tuesday morning. We were called out about two thirty a.m. and I've been sitting on Eastbourne Pier fully armed with my Platoon in position putting pennies in the slot machines ever since – It was rather fun being in command of a Pier – I had to resist the most enormous temptations like fishing or opening the Skittle Ball Alley, and it was magnificent not having to pay 2d to get on. I immediately commandeered the night watchman's bicycle – I'm probably one of the very few men who have bicycled up and down Eastbourne Pier in the moonlight of a night in May. I wished that you'd step out of a shadow and make love to me.

I love you so very much.

Always,

Tam

Tam to Margaret (postcard) Farnham, 28 May 1940

Suggest 'Always and Sometimes' as your theme song. Tam.

Tam to Margaret Eastbourne, Monday 4 June 1940

My Darling,

I couldn't telephone you at 1.15 today because I was wandering aimlessly about with a compass trying to find my way back here and when I finally did arrive at ten to two I only had threepence. I'm incredibly hot and disgustingly sticky – I should like one of those eau-de-cologne rubs you used to give me. Keep this quotation from George Santayana's[1] *Little Essays*. 'Nothing can be meaner than the anxiety to live on, to live on anyhow and in any shape; a spirit with any honour is not willing to live on except in its own way, and a spirit with any wisdom is not over eager to live at all.'

That is a pleasant and well-phrased truth and pleases me more than Mr Sassoon's[2] effort in the *Observer* yesterday – talking about 'future sunshine' and 'faith's front line' not in his old style at all, at all. I've got other horrible and difficult letters to write so I must say I love you and goodnight my sweet. Forever my darling,
Tam

1. George Santayana (1963–62), Spanish-born American philosopher and critic.
2. Siegfried Sassoon (1886–1967), poet.

Tam to Margaret Eastbourne, 14 June 1940

My Darling,

I'm afraid I was in poor form yesterday, I was tired and my brain was in a buzzing, bewildered muddle – half of every day now I hope I shan't be off until after the 24th and that until I do go I must make the most of everything, and the other half I'm cursing the Government of England for making such an appalling smudge in the pages of our history. It makes me rage and boil and feel sick when I pause to remember that Poland, Finland, and now France have been struck down and Great Britain has sunk the Graf Spee and had her army booted into the sea – the R.A.F. magnificent, I grant you – but it's horrible to hear France – with Paris fallen – screaming, literally screaming for help and to still see England swarming with troops – unequipped after ten months, untrained and useless. What an inadequate, inefficient and inglorious ally.

God Almighty how we've got to fight now to win back our reputation as a friend and how we've got to fight and die and fight again to get back our reputation as an enemy. It makes me sad and sore and black with misery – I knew Paris would fall – but now it has it is worse than I thought it was going to be. How can America refuse that last appeal of Reynaud's?[1] If it does I think the only corner left in all the world with any honour will be Finland and we shall have to learn the language and start a theatre in Helsinki. Oh Margaret, what a world we start our official lives together in.

I've been wondering for some weeks now if Democracy *is* the finest way a country can live – it seems to lead to such feeble-mindedness and unpreparedness and muddle and above all the cursed God damned bloody party politics. If America doesn't declare complete war you find the answer in the Presidential Election. The reason civilisation is in deadly peril is because of party politics – Atlee fighting conscription, Baldwin fighting re-armament, Chamberlain's policy of appeasement – party politics.

After this war perhaps we shall find a new system – somewhere between the iron rule and disregard of individualism of the Germans and the sloppy hopeless weakness of the English. You know how frightened I shall be and how tired and probably how useless when I do fight – but all today I've been longing for it. Instead I've been lying in a field in the sun drawing a map of a wood and it's driven me bloody well crazy. We ought to be pouring men into France, even if we have to send them in fishing boats and pleasure steamers and taxi cabs – as long as they've got rifles they ought to go. I admit the long view might be sacrifice France and establish a front further south – but if somebody's having their throat cut in the next room you don't turn out the light and go to sleep. Anyway it's not what I've been wearing shit-coloured suits for ten months for.

My darling you understand please,
Tam

1. Paul Reynaud (1878–1966), French President.

Margaret to Tam (telegram) London, (undated) 1940

SUGGEST YOU ORDER RING, STOP SULKING AND BE READY ON THE 21ST[1] STOP I LOVE YOU STOP

1. 21 June 1940 was their wedding day.

Tam to Margaret Eastbourne, 28 June 1940

My Darling,

Don't refer to my duty to my country as ratting on you – much as I adore digging up pleasure gardens, I prefer to have my lunch at the proper time, and in the old days of digging I always did, then I slept after lunch and then generally I had a picnic – but now I've got a pay parade. Longing for Sunday my pretty – but

how shall I wait all day until I get you on a bed? I have no money to post this. But I love you, Dear Mrs Williams.
Yours forever,
Dear Mr Williams.

Tam to Margaret — Eastbourne, 2 July 1940

Darling and Blessed Margaret,

Today has been full of flaps and foolishness and bugger Roumania. I don't like these dirty neutrals thinking we're beaten. See you soon but remember what I told you – take great care of yourself because you're enormously precious. My love to you my pretty,
Tam

Tam to Margaret — Eastbourne, 4 July 1940

My Darling and Valuable Margaret,

Thank you for your letter. Come down soon. Come down soon. Oh my sweet, life is so different when you're near. I feel such a gold digger asking you and cadging quids off you.

Oh Dear oh Dear, what about the Duke of Windsor, the crowning insult. 1936 King Emperor, 1940 Governor of the Bahamas, was there ever such a decline and fall? The finest Prince that Wales ever had and England's weakest King. Tragedy – big bold Greek stuff.

> 'Among our Ancient Mountains,
> Among our lonely dales,
> Oh let the prayer re-echo,
> God Bless the Governor of the Bahamas.'

There's a rumour we cancel our nightly stand-to from tomorrow for a bit – please God. Very wearying and the troops are hating it. My hair's full of dust and I've no money for a shampoo. Well, why shouldn't I hint?

No more except that I love you and I shall need you more and more as the world changes into something I have little interest in. Write to me my Beloved and please come here soon.
Forever and ever, Tamèd.

Tam to Margaret Eastbourne, 9 July 1940

My Darling,

Oh these trains going out of stations – they're like the end every time. Very weary today, just off to my little bed. Heard from Mother last night, she thinks it's essential Loo and Prue[1] go to America – in God's name how? She says there's an organisation by Actors for the evacuation of Actors' children.

I shan't be happy till I see you. Do something about it.

I love you so much,

Tam

1. Prudence, born in 1932, was Tam's second daughter by Gwynne Whitby.

Tam to Margaret Eastbourne, Thursday evening, 12 July 1940

My Darling,

You sounded rather worried and a little depressed when I spoke to you just now, as if half a bottle and a pleasing dinner and a beise[1] was what you needed. Someday my Margaret I shall not only diagnose but also effect the cure, until then – oh! the bravery we've got to summon up.

There's a scene in *Richard the Third*, one of Shakespeare's less subtle climaxes but nevertheless pretty God damned dramatic, Richard is about to be defeated by Richmond (the Earl not the suburb to you my Australian), his crown and his power which he gained by murder on the point of tumbling. He's asleep in his tent on the eve of battle and he dreams. The voices of the two little princes in the Tower whom he murdered, his wife Anne, Buckingham, Hastings and the Magnificent old Queen Margaret, all dead, torment him in his sleep and he wakes screaming and shrieking.

I, on the contrary, [am] at the moment innocent of murder, yet have voices hurting me on the eve of battle. They are the voices of bookmakers and waiters and croupiers and barmen. They shout the amounts I've lost and spent and thrown away and remind me – God wot not that I need it – that through my infamy my children and Gwynne[2] and my mother and my wife and her mother are all suffering unnecessary worry, hardship and unhappiness. This colourful confession all started with the word Bravery. For if I can overcome all of this, then – presuming I survive, prosper and repair my manifold weakness – then I shall not feel ashamed anymore.

At the moment I do, except when I'm too tired and too drunk. And I find and consider it brave to continue pursuing a direction and purpose feeling miserably and abjectly ashamed all the time. The last sentence is balls for I haven't the bloody alternative. To put it succinctly – am I worse than Mr Harrison?[3] Yes is the answer, for sacrifices should be made alone and not by one's womankind whose ages span some sixty years. All of which brings us back to the bookie, the waiter, the croup and the barman.

This my Darling is quite the most intimate letter I've ever written. You have my complete and naked thoughts, which is good in a way and may show you I love you more than I'm in love with you, for one conceals from one's lover what one can tell to the the one person in the world one really loves.

I hate your doing those bloody photographs.[4] I hate it. I hate cadging quids. I hate my darling daughters not having the protection they should, I hate Gwynne being harassed, worried and driven. I hate my sweet old devil Silver being kicked about in her old age and by God and all that's powerful I hate Mr Harrison – not because he's a rat and off to America to earn himself £10,000, but because his is the Bravery, the right kind of Bravery: 'To hell with what they think of me, I'm going to take care of myself and my own and later maybe I'll give England a hand' and mine is the weakness that said 'Oh I must join the bloody Army, everyone will say I'm a louse if I don't. Margaret won't love me and I'll feel a shit if I don't.'

I'm now going to have the most enormous whisky and then bed and sleep for eight precious hours. Forgive me for this miserable letter, it's more in anger than self-pity and I love you so. I love you so. Tamèd

1. Beise was a slang word for sex derived from the French verb 'baiser', to kiss.
2. Gwynne Whitby (1904–85), Tam's first wife.
3. Rex Harrison (1908–90, film and stage actor.
4. Margaret still did occasional work as a mannequin or model to earn extra money.

Tam to Margaret — Bexhill-on-Sea, Sunday evening, 5 July 1940

I always want to write to you the moment I've finished talking to you on the telephone. A sunny summer Sunday evening has reduced me to a state of severe sentimentality so when I've finished this I shall have a drink and probably a pull in the bath.

Sorry about that dreary letter my pretty, I shouldn't have posted it. But I can't talk to these good honest upright chaps here so I have to write to you. I wonder if there is such a thing as a cad in Bexhill-on-Sea? I think I'll advertise. 'Officer, public schoolboy, wishes to get in touch with a shit. Knowledge of racing, Baccarat, cheque-kiting, women and the theatre essential. Write:- 'Lonely' c/o Bexhill Argus.'

Oh my sweet I love you so desperately. I work and eat and sleep and read and wash and drink nowadays, and it all seems odd and funny somehow. I think of you nearly all the time, wondering how long it will be before we can taste for the first time together a normal existence. I'm beginning to get fearfully impatient with not being told who I really am. And I'm a little bit touchy that H.R.H. The Duke of Windsor has been given the Bahamas – they would have been so perfect for us.

Be happy my dearest Margaret, and be sweet to me. Write to me and love me. God bless you. Someday we'll take the Swastika dust sheet off the Georges V[1] and behave disgracefully again. I shall have the bidets filled with Gardenias and the bath with Ayala '28 and you with happiness. Till then I remain your loving husband, 2nd Lieutenant H.A.G. Williams (6898874) 8th Bn. Devonshire Regt.

1. One of their favourite haunts in Paris was the Georges Cinq Hotel.

Tam to Margaret Bexhill-on-Sea, 16 July 1940

Margaret my Darling,

Very weary, so only a note. Has your little Mummy got herself a gas mask yet? I think she should at once and is yours working alright? *You should always carry them now*. I'm not trying to frighten you my pretty, it's just that they might use it and you'd feel such a fool in Shaftesbury Avenue in a gas bombardment with your respirator in Chelsea. A tragedy happened last night, one of my china teeth fell out off the back. Saw the dentist today, I told him if he couldn't fix it for half a guinea I'd fill it up with chewing gum till after the war.

Forever my Darling, Tamèd

Tam to Margaret Bexhill-on-Sea, Wednesday 18 July 1940

If you, but for this war, would be the happiest wife in all the world, then I Madam, would be the happiest man, the most adoring husband and the most ardent lover.

You know what to do with the enclosed I trust.
Travel on them towards me.

Tam to Margaret London, 24 July 1940

My Darling and Most Lovely Margaret,

Thank you my angel for £3. Mrs Cargill insisted on only charging me 18/- which is really amazingly cheap. I paid her the £1 of my other debts and dined at the Café Royal on the change which was 4/6 and went to *Pinochio* which I adored. I've known Sir Jiminy so very intimately for years it was pleasant to actually see and hear him, the dear little nuisance. What a genius Disney is to make a loveable character out of a conscience, of all beastly unattractive material. The whole thing was very 'Peer Gynt' I thought.

Off to the dentist now, had a bit of a toothache this week. I never have the bloody toothache till I go to the dentist. They give it to you so you have to go back to them.

Take care of yourself my sweet. Forever and ever, Tamèd

Tam to Margaret Bexhill-on-Sea, 24 July 1940

My Beloved,

The wind isn't blowing and the sun is shining, but because you've gone the day and the evening seem dull and lonely. It was such heaven having you here, just to feel your whereabouts was near.

I seem to have got some nice blokes on the course, but only one of them appears to be able to shoot. It's a change and I think I'll enjoy my week.

I'll try and never write depressing letters my pretty. You said I sometimes did yesterday, but if they sometimes are you'll have to understand and forgive me. I get so lonely and so bored.

My love to you and thank you for coming, Tamèd

P.S. Please could you make the end of the war 1941, and do you think we could afford two cars in Australia? I'd like something vulgar of my very own and you could have something in black.

Tam to Margaret Bexhill-on-Sea, 25 July 1940

A year ago today we sat on a rock in the golden glory of a warm sun and bathed in a sea as blue as God's heaven. We ate peaches and green almonds and white caprecau cheese and bread and radishes and drank rough cheap strong wine cooled in the pools and in the evening sun we were rowed from our rock to where a very old carriage and a rather old horse pulled us up the steep hill to the top of the Island.[1]

Later we dined and drank and a handsome Prince appeared and we quarrelled. How could we have quarrelled you may ask, but we did and no love was made when love should have been made.

Today, heavily clothed and burdened with several hundred things hanging round my neck, the rain from heaven mingled with the sweat of my body and I had for my companions fifteen Devon Dumplings. No peaches, no wine, no carozza, no white cheese, no green almonds, no blue sea, no radishes, no warm rock, no magic Island, no Margaret.

Don't let's ever quarrel again.

I adore you too much. Tamèd

1. In 1939 Tam pawned his mother's mink coat for £67 in order to take Margaret on holiday to Capri.

Tam to Margaret

Bexhill-on-Sea, Saturday evening,
Orderly Ape, 6 August 1940

How sweet you were on the telephone. Hell and Darkness! How cruel is that bloody instrument, to hear only, not to touch, not to see, only to hear. Agony. Scientists don't understand lovers. They invent beastly nasty things to hurt them. All the old busybodies get over-excited about traps that break little animals and write to the R.S.P.C.A. – why isn't there a R.S.P.T.L.? Royal Society for the Prevention of Torture to Lovers. It's a scandal. They're at me again. This time with another of their filthy contrivances, the radio. 'Parlez moi D'amour' A lover is more easily hurt than the tiniest sweetest little mouse and yet nobody does anything.

OH dear OH dear OH dear, to hear only.

'Every little cat and dog and crawling thing may look on her, but Romeo may not'

Next week my Darling, Thursday my Darling, I want you so badly. On Thursday you shall quench me. No hearing only, seeing, touching, feeling.

Goodnight Beloved, God Bless you. Be good and love me.

Forever my Pretty, Tam.

Tam to Margaret Bexhill-on-Sea, Monday 6 August 1940

'The Artist lives a lonely, miserable life at the best of times. His trade is difficult, he only wants to do the best and he never reaches the best; he is solitary, he is impatient and bad-tempered and full of sadness; and he is madly gay to escape the shadows. But – and it is a supreme But – he is endowed by God with one gift that saves all. He knows the secret of the world as human beings have to live it. He knows there is no life, no happiness, no misery, no ecstacy, nor suicide, nor great work, nor exquisite beauty, without women. Women are the Light of the World to poor, small ignorant men.'

That, my little pocket Venus, must have been written by a man who loved a woman and I have taken great trouble to copy it out so that you may read it, because it is beautifully written. Not, as you already suppose, because I wished you to imagine that such were my feelings for you.

You're too confident, too vain. I doubt if I shall tell you again I adore and worship you until our silver wedding day. I've been sitting underneath my bloody bandstand, in a sandbagged room stinking of mildew and foulness for twelve and a half hours. A curious way of doing one's duty. It's some divisional exercise which has obviously developed into a complete Military balls up and I and my dumplings have long since been forgotten. If you don't see me on Thursday, look for me here.

God Bless you my Darling, you'll make the Islands of Scilly more beautiful for me by standing on them.

TAMÈD

Tam to Margaret Bexhill-on-Sea, Wednesday evening, 7 August 1940

My Darling,

If Adolf isn't exceptionally and wilfully stupid I shall be with you nice and early tomorrow, but the nearer it gets to seeing you and feeling free for a week, the more convinced I am that our Island Fortress may be assailed and my Leave cancelled for ever. We're standing to from 2.30 in the morning and working straight on till lunchtime, like we used to.

Ask Wilfred[1] to drink with me at the Green Room and then we'll give your little Mum a fat little grouse and a bottle of Claret – oh what magic words. I couldn't be more excited if we were landing in New York in an hour. What a lot of money I shall spend on your clothes when I'm rolling in money again. I'm as randy as a red hot panther. TAMÈD

1. Wilfrid Hyde-White (1903–91), actor and supreme gambling companion.

Tam to Margaret Bexhill-on-Sea, Sunday 18 August 1940

My Darling,

What a lovely day. A week ago we were bumping about and you were catching two mackerel and I was catching four. I've been in the most awful miasma of depression since I returned. I suppose it's the inevitable reaction after a week of happiness. It's curious that I still think that the days with you are my real life and the Army is just something barely endurable that is not at all real.

I spent yesterday reading the most disturbing little volume ever written, called *Guilty Men* – you remember I've been wanting it. It says quite plainly that since 1923 we have been governed without any judgement or honesty or honour or reason or foresight, by a collection of utterly corrupt old men, who, as they decay or become too brazenly dishonest, are sent off to the House of Lords. In fact our House of Lords has become the Twentieth Century's Botany Bay. I beg your pardon, I forgot for the moment I was addressing my wife, none other than Australia's premier Ambassaddress [*sic*] of Beauty. Dear God! 'If England were what England seems and not the England of our dreams'. Duff Cooper[1] emerges as the one man with honour, a poet, a gentleman, scrupulous and brave. He *must* govern Post War England, there is no one else.

God wot me for a fool. Am I writing a lover's letter to Duff Cooper or to my own most adorable wife whom I adore and worship and long for, whom I shall pamper and cherish and spoil, on whom I shall shower the comforts and pleasures of life, with whom I shall enjoy such enormous happiness and tremendous fun. Oh my Darling I love you. Take care of every inch of yourself and behave properly,

Always and always, Tamèd

1. Sir Alfred Duff Cooper (1890–1954), later Viscount Norwich of Aldwick. Resigned his post of First Lord of the Admiralty after the appeasement of Hitler at Munich as the terms 'stuck in his throat'.

Tam to Margaret Bexhill-on-Sea, Monday 26 August 1940

My Darling,

I couldn't hear a word you said on the phone this morning. You were too sleepy and last night was such a hurried 'My regiment sails at dawn' kind of goodbye, but thank you for coming down and reminding me that life is lovely and love magnificent.

God what a day. I'm absolutely dead shagged flat beat. When I undressed even my tie was soaking and so much salt sweat had run into my eyes that they were bloodshot. I kept on thinking why didn't I sit down more all those years before I was in the Army – in fact why did I ever stand up? Get going with your book. Now is the time before the smell of Paris is out of your nostrils and the world is so changed that it is an effort to remember the days that were different. Never forget that we're terribly lucky to have seen Monte Carlo and Paris and the Riviera as they were, wonderful and gay, as they may never be again. The longer I live I realise that, after providing for those you're responsible for, the next most important thing is to squeeze and knock and press and scratch happy moments, happy days and holidays for oneself. 'The days that make us happy make us wise.' I think without knowing it you've always realised that. And starting from scratch you've done amazingly. *That's* why your life is interesting and you have character. The reasons that will make your own story interesting.[1]

Tell the little man to keep you the blue Bristol, I'll give it to you. But are you sure the stuff is Bristol, it sounds incredibly cheap. Are you fond of coloured glass, I'm not quite sure. I suppose in my own home I wouldn't mind it, in other people's I always suspect that it conceals the weakness of a drink.

I must totter to the Mess and find whisky, but it won't taste as good as some water from a well that a farm woman gave me this afternoon.

God bless you, may your heart always be doing lovely things[2] and let me be in your heart always, I love you so much, Tam

1. No evidence survives to suggest that Margaret ever made significant headway with writing her autobiography.
2. Quoting from 'Her Heart' by John Masefield.

Tam to Margaret Bexhill-on-Sea, Wednesday 28 August 1940

Darling,

Your letter revived a flagging spirit. Nineteen miles today including a battle. Six miles in an hour and ten minutes, full equipment, only two of my little fellows gave in and fell by the way, not bad. Their aged Platoon Commander was what in happier days and places we called 'under the whip'. I had one moment of feeling the biggest shit in the world. I told them they could pinch some apples from an orchard, no sooner said than done. Five minutes later the woman who owned the orchard offered us tea, cake and at least four lbs of apples and plums. She brewed the tea and just as it was ready we had to move on. What must she think of human nature on this lovely summer evening. I wish I could take her out to dinner and try to explain.

Very very fatigued my darling – I'd give a lot for a massage and a bottle and dinner in bed – oysters and a cold grouse and you in a dressing gown. Forever, provided I last, TAMÈD

P.S. Those very ugly feet of mine behaved quite decently. Just had a foot inspection – I prefer the more conservative type of aperitif.

Tam to Margaret Bexhill-on-Sea, Monday 2 September 1940

My Darling

In my youth I became accustomed to getting out of warm beds, and finding a taxi I would make my way home. I didn't like it then, but now I'm older and respectably married to a wife I adore most passionately, still to have to jump out at three in the bloody morning and bicycle (a bloody broken bicycle) two miles up hill in pitch black out is my new low in misery. But my Darling, you come and go (or perhaps I should say come come come come come come come come come come come come come and go) and you make me happy while you're here and when you leave I remember how lovely you are and then I look forward to your coming back and that's all the happiness there is in life. All the rest is boredom and discomfort and physical exertion and bad food eaten in deplorable company. So that my philosophy tells me that it's better to jump out of a warm bed at three in the bloody morning etc etc. than to have no warm bed to get into in the first place.

Do you think it would be nice if we both gave me a wedding present? Will you telephone your Mr Cecil Beaton[1] and ask him

what his price is. Tell him we're broke and the only picture I have of you is on the cover of *Woman's Own*. I think he may be cheap at the moment and not very busy. Will you enquire please? A little good news. We leave on Sunday to start our nomad gypsying excursion through Sussex – we sleep in dew drenched fields under the moon and stars and I shall be Queen of the May. I shall be the most pissed Queen of the May you ever saw and I shall read again Davies'[2] *Autobiography of a Super-Tramp*, a book you ought to read, and his poems, they're good. Then we shall return like John the Baptist from his locusts and wild honey in the wilderness for Thursday, Friday, Saturday and Sunday of next week, which would mean no hopping out of a warm bed. Give my love to my little blue mother, telephone Cecil Beaton, get me out of the Army, take care of yourself, love me incessantly, send me my lighter, start your autobiography, go to bed early and I'll promise not to smell the next time you come come come come come come come come come come down.
I really do adore you, Tam

1. Cecil Beaton (1904–80), photographer, designer, portrait artist. He *did* paint a portrait of Margaret, but sometime after the war.
2. W.H. Davies (1871–1940), Welsh poet.

Tam to Margaret

Bexhill-on-Sea, Friday evening,
7 September 1940

Friday evening, time was when Friday evening meant eighty pounds, eighty sovereigns, eighty bloody quid for eight performances. It takes me five long months to earn eighty quid now – September, October, November, December, January.

Ha Ha Ha! Hee Hee Hee!!!
Little brown jug and a Big Watney.

Three letters from you today my Darling. Poor little red-eyed hag I feel so sorry for you and long to cure your cold in the only proper and pleasing manner. A cracking dinner, a quantity of wine of a good quality and so to bed to complete the treatment. The next morning the cold is gone and you are merely hungover and pregnant.

Once again the Army is having its fun. They prepare us for a three days' march, but it's only a passing whim, they change their frivolous little minds, they were only teasing after all. 'Oh you great big Tease Major General' and now not only do we not march, we don't even bloody well walk outside the gate!

There's another flap on – the moon is up or the tide is out or Churchill's finished his cigar. I give up. We're all confined to billets and I'm left with little gargantua to be permanent orderly officer until further notice. 'The fault, dear Brutus, is not in our stars but in ourselves that we are Orderlies'. I'm a little light-headed I fancy, the Army's got me, I'm nuts. Perhaps not really, perhaps only in terrible need of you and Peace. I love you so much, so dearly and so well.
Goodnight Beloved, Tam

P.S. Darling, can you send me a quid? I've paid my debts off and I haven't a bob and if the flap stops and we go off on Wednesday or so for this march I shall need some of them. Sorry, sorry, sorry.

Tam to Margaret Bexhill-on-Sea, Thursday evening (undated)

My Darling,

Telephoning has been quite impossible. Nothing but chocolate since my bacon and eggs, it's been one Titanic M.F.U. [Major Fuck Up], quite, quite monstrous, but tonight we balanced up a little. Exceedingly tired after this enormous journey, I'm a little confused as to whether it is the Thames or the Mississippi that we cross tomorrow. My love to Jasmine[1] the darling, and to you my sweet. I'll telephone when I can, here are the railway things. I must sleep.
God bless you and I adore you, Tamèd

1. Jasmine Bligh (1913–91), Margaret's great friend, a niece of the Earl of Darnley and one of the BBC's first television announcers when the service opened in 1936. Married to Sir John Paley Johnson but in love with General John 'Sandy' Lane.

She Nodded and Said that She Would

We met, then your flowers arrived with a note,
'Seventy-two red roses aren't nearly enough,' you wrote,
'So I'm bringing some orchids round at nine,
The orchids and I wish to take you to dine.'
I tried to telephone some excuse, no good,
I laughed and I nodded and said that I would.

A kiss in a taxi and I fell into love
As the stars kissed the morning high up above.
Promises given and promises sworn
Strangers at midnight were lovers by dawn.
The moment I saw you I knew that we should,
That's why I nodded and said that I would.

Music. The scent of Lilac. The choir boys in white,
A stained glass window stencilling the light.
Singing, then silence, and a voice began
Calmly, dispassionately, 'Will you take this man'.
With love in my heart beside you I stood
And trembled and nodded and said that I would.

You chose the Ritz to kiss my heart goodbye
Crowded at lunchtime, so that I couldn't cry,
You were in love with someone else and wanted a divorce
You said 'I'll send you evidence and make a settlement of
  course'.
You asked if I'd consent and if I understood
And once more I nodded and said that I would.[1]

1. This poem was written by Tam and slipped into a letter without remark.

Tam to Margaret — Sunday evening (undated)

My Darling,

I hope to heaven you heard and saw little of that bloody raid last night. I've missed you so much this weekend, if the flap is over next week will you come down please? I shall try and telephone you after seven if that bloody siren doesn't blow off. . . That was written last night and of course I tried to telephone but couldn't. I shall try again now as soon as the raid has passed. I'm getting very worried about you and think if it's *possible* you must get out of London. It's getting bad and it drives me mad wondering how you are and if you've been frightened. I know it's probably perfectly alright but today I've been in a complete state of jitters about it. The posts are all delayed and we get no papers till late in the afternoon. Darling do try and go somewhere, here if possible and where cheaper? If not somewhere out of London. I'm certain the raids will intensify and that Hitler's trying his bloodiest to finish the war before the winter by dropping everything he can on us and

London is going to be his main objective. I love you my darling Margaret and you're to do as you're told.
Forever, Tamèd

Tam to Margaret — Lutterworth, Friday evening, 1 November 1940

This is getting more and more boring. Lutterworth – OH MY. John Wycliffe who translated the Bible lived here and they water the ink in the Post Office. That's all I shall ever know about Lutterworth. Tomorrow we reach the Rockies.[1] I miss you simply terribly. Are you taking care of yourself? Be ready to leave by Tuesday.
My love to you all from a young fellow in Lutterworth.

1. Tam frequently ironically compared the unit at this time to pioneering frontiersmen.

Tam to Margaret — Lincoln, Tuesday 10 December 1940

My Darling,

Thank you for your sweet note waiting for me last night. I spent the day hobbling about and decided that as they're over the fields and turnips today I'd malinger a little and remain here. So I've just finished reading all the morning papers. I can't tell you what *will* happen, but I'll tell you what *might* happen. Italy I really think will collapse, completely collapse. And as far as we're concerned it doesn't matter if Hitler takes over Italy or lets Mussolini stew in his own juice. Any big move Hitler makes in the Balkans will be met with a war with Russia and Turkey. I think Russia will go to war with Germany. I think the Italian African Empire will no longer be in existence in a year and the War will certainly be over any time between April 1941 and September 1942. This new drive in Egypt is just the very thing that was needed. I really feel we're winning and after all the defeats and failures and muddles of six months ago[1] why the bloody hell the Press aren't shouting it from the house tops I can't imagine. England is supposed never to know when she is beaten, but that's no reason why she shouldn't know when she's winning. It makes me so ANGRY.

Darling don't go anywhere without letting me know and for God's sake take care of your precious self. My love to our Mums and so much to you my lovely and adorable and very valuable wife,
Forever, Tam

P.S. Don't forget my embarrassing inability to leave Lincoln. I've borrowed 2/-

1. The evacuation from Dunkirk, 4 June 1940.

Margaret to Tam

The Berkeley Hotel, London,
Saturday (undated) 1940

My own beloved,

I'm becoming the leading Berkeley borrower, always use their notepaper. Well now, the film[1] looks even more definite than before. Today they asked for confirmation in writing that I had agreed to make the picture, and they want a photographic test on Wed morning, so I shall return to you on Wed eve a slightly richer woman *I hope I hope I hope*.

Oh dear how did you manage about paying your mess bill at Lincoln? Darling you know I would never let you down if I could possibly help it – but I hadn't a penny. I'd miscalculated somehere and left myself badly in the soup. I pray we are able to land this picture otherwise once more we are up the well known creek.

I feel a bit of an ass rushing out of London each evening but it costs very little and I do sleep. The guns, if not the bombs, make such a noise. So have just been working hard and *no parties*. But now as I have to stay till Wed I'm going to do some photographic work.
Darlingest miss me every moment of the day, and pray for me too.
My love to Silver,
God bless you always and always,
I adore you, Your M.

1. Margaret is probably referring to the film *Dangerous Comment* in which she did succeed in getting a part.

Tam and Margaret

Bexhill-on-Sea, Friday evening,
29 December 1940

Here's 'Bottle Party Lullaby', pretty damned good too, I'll settle for a pound.

An amazing spectacle this evening, as none of the troops could go out we persuaded the Band to come and play to us at about six. In the middle an air-raid warning went. And there was the band on the cricket pitch, on this lovely summer evening, long shadows on the grass and the sun sinking and reflecting in the windows, with their tin hats on and eye shields and gas capes, playing a selection from the 'Maid of the Mountains' as full of memories of the last War as a casualty list in *The Times*. Macdonald, Baldwin, Chamberlain, the whole bloody gang of them have made suckers out of all of us. But it was a strange sight, sad and stimulating and strange and one that Mr Sassoon would have made a pretty song about.

Bottle Party Lullaby

Debutantes in celebration
Dowagers in perspiration
Dancing, to the drone
Of sex and saxaphone.
Gigolo with resignation
Hired blondes beyond salvation
Laughing, dancing to their doom
In this syncopated tomb.

Stars and stoogies congregate here
Rakes and roués dissipate here
Come and buy us all a drink
Join the sty and all its stink.
Floosies, freaks and flageotists,
Misers, morons, masochists
Coloured men and columnists
Toughs and tarts and titles mix
Membership is seven and six.

Conga, Ragtime Swing and Rumba
Striptease and a dirty number
Entertain the clientele
To a Cabaret in a padded cell –
Lovelies find their lovers with 'em
Drunk with passion, wine and rhythm
Dancing with a desperation
To this sepulchre of syncopation.

Bankrupts and the Bankers meet here
Baronets and Bookies meet here
All escaping, dancing, drinking
Hurrying away from thinking.
Pansies, Peers and Pugilists,

Chorus-girls and capitalists
Millionaire mysogonists,
Jail-birds, Jurors, Judges mix,
Membership is seven and six.

Tam to Margaret Margate, (undated) 1940

Twenty years ago I toiled round Margate searching for my first threatrical rooms. When I found them, the bed from the previous occupant had not been made and there was the remains of a large melon on the washing stand. I hurried to the theatre to see my name in print and to my shattering disappointment, opposite the character I was playing, who was called Tim Bradbury, was the name Walter Plinge. No Hugh Williams. Walter Plinge. And after the performance I was given the sack. However, by the time we arrived at Deal for the last three nights of the week I had improved and they kept me on. I was so delighted I bought a Fox Terrier which nobody liked and proved a fearful handicap in looking for lodgings so I gave him to Gwynne who immediately gave it to somebody else. It was a lovely hot summer and I earned four pounds a week and saved £1. The stage was nicer in those days. No films – no agents to speak of – and there were such lovely actors – Ainley[1] and Gerald[2] and Hawtrey[3] and Fay Compton[4] and the Ballet really was the Ballet. How odd that I'm looking for billets again today and that my salary is 3s less a week than in 1921.

Forgive me darling I'm meandering on like Dame Mary herself – to hell with 1921, it was a wonderful champagne year which has all been drunk now and let's leave it at that. 1961 is what matters and the years of fun till then. Little disgusting will have finished school – we shall be living in sunshine and solvency, you'll be elegant and lovely with the blueness of your eyes wandering towards brown young men on the beach. . . But I expect to see you before that. Take care of your precious self, you're very valuable.
Always and always,
Tam

1. Henry Ainley, actor of the old school, died 1945.
2. Gerald Du Maurier (1873–1934), actor and playwright, father of novelist Daphne Du Maurier.
3. Sir Charles Hawtrey, actor, died 1923.
4. Fay Compton (1894–1978) actress.

Waiting for Midnight, December 31st 1940

Goodbye Old Year. Most hated and abhor'd of all the Years
This World has ever known.
And yet to me, most blessed and adored
Because you leave me Margaret for mine own.

There follows a gap in the correspondence during 1941 and into 1942 as Tam was released from the army to make a series of morale-boosting films such as One of Our Aircraft is Missing, Secret Mission, Ships with Wings, Talk about Jacqueline *and* The Day will Dawn *at the Denham Studios in England, with the well-known team of Michael Powell and Emeric Pressburger. During this time Margaret gave birth to their son Hugo. In July 1942 Tam returned to the Devonshire Regiment and was based in South-West England.*

The following poem (undated) is one of the half-dozen or so that Tam wrote during the war and sent to Margaret.

I am not fighting for the Poles or Czechs,
And – only indirectly for the Rex:
I do not greatly love the Slav or Greek,
I cannot bear the way Colonials speak.
I loathe efficiency and Nissen huts,
And as for Bonhomie I hate its guts.
I am not fighting Germans just to get
My democratic share of 'blood and sweat'.
Dear Sir I feel that you may get the gist,
Of all my war-time aims from the following list:-
Georgian houses, real replicas of Heaven,
Split pediments, breakfast at eleven;
Large white peonies in big white bowls,
Aspargus 'au beurre', white bait in shoals,
A sunny breakfast froom, a library with books,
An English butler, one or two French cooks;
Clean white housemaids in new print frocks,
Coachmen turned chauffers, footmen on the box;
Dinner parties all in evening dress;
Glamorous women drenched in 'Mary Chess',
Charades and paper games; hot houses with the heat on;
Superficiality and Cecil Beaton;
Shrimps from Morcambe Bay, port that is tawny;
Claret and Beaujolais, soles that are 'Mornay';
Hot scones for tea, thick cream, the smell of logs,
Long country walks, thick shoes and spaniel dogs,
Ducks in the evening, swishing swans in flight,
Fires in bedrooms flickering at night,
And of those 'Autrefois', all those 'moeurs',
Which are epitomised in 'Valse des Fleurs',
Fresh shiny chintzes, a herbaceous border, . . .
Death and destruction to the damned 'New Order'.

Tam to Margaret Sunday morning (undated), 1942

My Darling,

I came here purposely to try and telephone you this morning, but the Commanding Officer is in the vicinity so can't risk a personal call on H.M. telephone. So instead I've been signing my name incessantly for over an hour on innumerable bits of ridiculous forms. How are you my sweet? How's your cough? Did the Blitz worry you on Friday night? Are you taking care of yourself? And do you love me? To all these I want answers so badly. I miss you enormously as you can well imagine and I loathe the thought that you may be frightened.

How's the picture[1] and is there anyone pleasant or amusing on it? Is Mr Mason[2] attractive and are you happy and when do you think you'll come back to me – I want you so badly my love.

I must go. Love me please and come up as soon as you possibly can and in less than three weeks we shall be alone. After the war when I dress beautifully and smell nice again and live a life that's tolerable, I shall be gay again and glamorous and no longer just a rather tedious husband. Until then have patience my pretty and kind wife, have patience.

Forever my love,
Tam

1. *The Young Mr Pitt*, directed by Carol Reed, released in 1942.
2. James Mason (1909–87), film star.

Margaret to Tam Welwyn Studios, Herts, 1942

Tam darling one,

I just wanted you to know I arrived safely. Bloody awful trip, however it was a fairly easy day's work. James Mason is not at all bad looking, but methinks a little wet. However he is happily married and so am I!! And the other people look rather alike to me so far, but they all know you and send their love. As I came home tonight the sky over London was bright pink for a radius of what looked like miles and miles and miles. Oh dear, how angry it makes me when I actually see this sort of thing, and yet we go on quoting to each other 'To the death'. What does it mean? Surely there have been enough deaths and enough hearts broken and homes smashed and enough talking done by the men who rule us. Let us have done! Hark at me!

I my darling not only send ALL of my very best love, but all of my heart my love. Always and always, your M.

Margaret to Tam Welwyn Studios, Herts, 1942

Oh my darling,

A hundred things a day happen to make me miss you more and more and hope and pray that one day we need never be apart.

There is absolutely no news, as nothing happens here except film making. I've been working very hard every day since I came here. Then we all go out to dinner together, I have several mild and bitters and hope to be in bed by 9.30 or 10.

Mum says you are working hard, she also said you were very good at the concert, but I want to know more. Did you do Henry V's speech? And how was it? I did want to get there but I finished on Sat afternoon and was called first thing Monday morning. Impossible to make it.

Tamèd, your New Year's poem made me cry. What a lucky girl I am to have your love and how careful I shall be to keep it always. Will know by tomorrow when I shall finish and will write immediately, but they are re-taking the end and are a bit behind schedule. However, I've done the ten days so now the more the merrier.
God bless you my beloved,
Always and always my love
Your own M.

P.S. You are up for a picture, very interested indeed.

Tam to Margaret Sidmouth, Tuesday 21 July 1942

Well well, here we are in OHaag VIII B. But I'd better start at the beginning. After a journey on the floor of the Guards Van I arrived at Torquay, reported and was booted off here. Back via Exeter once again where I dined, very dejectedly, in the bay window of the Clarence listening to church singing round the corner and watching the candelabras in the Cathedral swinging in the breeze through the blitzed windows. Exeter had a sort of tranquil hang-over, from the raids. The place is quite certainly the end, the bottom, a new low. I feel very well aware that I'm not really ideally situated for grumbling, having just had the happiest year of my life, but it is quite ghastly, the troops simply frightful, all low category, shit order and hopelessly slack. And the Officers – Dear God.

I couldn't write yesterday, not that I hadn't time, there's plenty of time, time is one of the big enemies. I had one of my days of panic. Complete and utter terror that I couldn't pull myself together. I had one at the beginning of the War, one in the summer of 1927 somewhere near St Malo, and a couple at school. I was really so miserable I had the quite certain knowledge that I should never be happy again and the hope was gone. Today I've written to Andrew Lawrence and he vaguely said he might get me a job. For this, apart from all the rest, is not a job for anybody under eighty.

No more, the post is waiting. I'll write more later this evening. SO much to say about loving you. Don't tell Hugo I've been grumbling or anyone else. My love to him and you,
Always and always my darling.

Margaret to Tam — Halfway Cottage, Dorney, Nr Windsor, 22 July 1942

My Beloved,

I'm just going to drop you a note tonight then add to it tomorrow. Got my identity card this morning, and sat for Nora[1] today. She has decided to call the picture Jasmine, because it is growing in the arch behind me!!! I'm not mad about it yet. Who is Andrew Lawrence and what kind of job can he get you? Have you given up the idea of the Phantoms?

Today I went to the British Restaurant. Oh dear what a sweaty crush. I served fifty eight full lunches and got one sixpenny tip. I did not know what to say! So I looked meek and said Thank you Sir. At 2.30 we sat down for spam and marg. How I longed for you and a drink but they were shut. So I did my weekly shopping and came home laden in the bus to our boy, what heaven he is. At 10 o'clock at night he seems to miss you almost as much as I do – his big eyes wander about the room looking for his dark, funny-smelling Daddy. Am I being foolish?

Thursday 23rd

Oh my darling, your letter arrived this morning, how I wish I were with you, what a hell hole it must be. I can't even find Sydmouth [*sic*] on my bloody map, where exactly are you from Exeter? I had

a feeling you were having a lousy trip. What a nostalgic dinner you must have had in Exeter. Remember?
Darling, remember our 'Over the Hill' and 'You and Me Together Love'. I have to and do always.

1. Nora Cundell, artist, the sister of Margaret's friend Vi Eaton.

Tam to Margaret Devon, Wednesday 22 July 1942

My Darling,

I felt so mean for writing such a depressive letter yesterday, a great deal of it was remorse. I feel bloody now for spending such an absurd amount of money in the last ten days. We only drank far too much and didn't have nearly so much fun or beising in consequence. However I shall, even I, have considerable difficulty in spending more than a £1 a week here. There isn't a single house in sight and only two buses a week pass the gate, no Mess, we have troops' food and I haven't had a drink since Sunday.

I inquired today if the troops had done any bayonet fighting. 'Yes we did a bit Sir,' a Sergeant told me. 'We did have two sandbag targets but them old cows in the field there ate up all the hay in them, since then we haven't bothered really'. Very boring but it shows the form.

I spend a lot of hours thinking of Halfway Cottage and the precious people in it and how wonderfully happy I've been there and how much I love you and how grateful I am. Life after the War always seemed as if it would be very sweet and now we know a little how sweet, indeed, it could be. I thought of you last night doing Hugo, wondering if that look in your eyes was there 'I've done it, I've managed, very well in fact, but now I want a drink, quickly please'. Oh my darling Margaret, how I love you. Compensations here include – lovely views, larks, and I imagine an occasional bathe with those in the Company not too infirm to venture.

God bless, write when you can, I miss you every minute all the time,
Always and always,
Tam

Tam to Margaret Sidmouth, Thursday 23 July 1942

My Beloved,

A letter from you this morning.[1] Sidmouth with an 'I' is some thirty miles from Torquay, eighteen from Exeter. Weekends are no good and it'd be pointless you staying for more than a night. I'll find some little place on the coast and we'll meet there, Exeter as I said is sorrowfully bruised and quiet.

I saw the M.O.[2] yesterday. He looked like a call boy and had a twitch in his eye. He said he'd try and fix the Aldershot Hospital[3] but was afraid it would be Exeter; but now my memory has been refreshed regarding the speed of Army methods, it will be three months come mucking day before anything happens. My spirits are rising with the course of the war, which is simply the same thing as saying my faith in Russia was a little shaken and now restored. On No 1 Court Auckinleck and Rommell are having an interesting battle,[4] but it is on the Centre Court with Bock and Timoshenko that the whole thing will be decided.[5] Obvious observation. Quite.

Prudie in her letter to me this morning said 'I did love that day we had on the Hill and I love you, OH I do'. That was the day that fixed her.[6] It really is very wonderful I think.

No more now darling – hope to telephone you this evening. Go on being wonderful to me for always and always,
Tam

1. This letter appears to have arrived the day it was sent. It may be an example of Margaret's habit of post-dating letters that Tam often complained about.
2. Medical Officer.
3. Tam needed surgery for a torn cartilage.
4. The Middle East campaign.
5. The Russian Marshal S.K. Timoshenko suffered a punishing defeat at the hands of the Germans in Kharkov.
6. The day that cemented her relationship with Tam.

Tam to Margaret Sidmouth, Monday morning, 27 July 1942

My Darling,

Thank you for your letter this morning and the chocolate, my God it's like being at school isn't it? My mum sent me chocolates this morning! One day I shall wake with a very sore bottom and find it's 1917.

Well, I'm off to somewhere that the hermits here tell me is pretty lonely, in contradistinction to this hub of the universe. I shall be on my own entirely, but apparently get relieved for twenty four hours every week in case the strain snaps your hair and you jump off the cliff. So that you'll be able to come down next week just the same but not to Lyme Regis but to Exmouth. Keep your sixpenny tip darling, I'd like it on one of my props.[1] I must go and see to my packing darling, will let you know tomorrow or Wednesday what the new joint is like. Don't care for the news, except the strengthening of Hitler's SS Waffen Troops, his own body guard, which he's now building up to the strength of an army. What we should call working up to an exit. My love to my son and to you my Beloved all my other love for always and always. Yes by Golly! You and me together love. But life has always been to me either very good or almost impossible. Next time it's very good we must invent a word to mean the opposite of grumble, and having invented it we must use it frequently. Not that I think we've taken our spasmodic happiness for granted, have we?

Write often my lovely Margaret,

Tam

1. After the war Tam had the sixpence set into his lighter.

Tam to Margaret Sidmouth, Tuesday 28 July 1942

Darling,

I do hope I see you soon. Next week. I walked into Budleigh last night, and with unerring instinct (perfected by practice) located a very nice bar in a very nice Hotel. It soon filled up with a lot of Royal Marine Officers, very jolly and young with a most magnificent Colonel who was stinking. They recognised me and couldn't have been nicer and invited me to dine on Thursday, so I felt considerably cheered up. I found an old Sergeant from the 8th here who lives in the neighbourhood who appeared overjoyed to see me and inquired at once when you were coming down, promised to fix rooms for you, get eggs and cream for me, arrange with the Farmer for me to shoot over his fields and for the Pro at the Golf Club to lend me some clubs. There's practically no work to do and anyway I feel by comparison enormously efficient.

Don't like the Russian news much, though of course they had Rostov before and it can't be easy fighting always against the clock as well as your adversary.[1] I see Churchill has postponed his statement on the course of the War until after the Summer recess – Why?

How's my Hugo, I think of you both so much my darlings – apart from loving you I am so very proud of you. I'm going to thank God for my *Times* subscription here – I'm stuck here now till Thursday evening. God bless you my precious, I'll let you know which nights next week,
Forever and ever. Always and always, Tam

1. Since the first defeat for Germany in the Russian campaign, when they were beaten at Rostov on 29 November 1941, Hitler had been cutting a swathe through Russian defences. The fall of Sebastopol on 1 July 1942 prepared the way for an advance on Stalingrad but any significant fighting had to be completed before the onset of the Russian winter.

Tam to Margaret Sidmouth, Thursday 30 July 1942

My Darling,

My Sergeant tells me – he has what are known as connections, that Straight Deal, Treasure from Heaven and Here's Hoping are good for Windsor on Saturday. I shall have three cross doubles (£1), will you phone Connie's and tell them to place the bet. Have a good day my darling. How I wish I were going with you. We had fun the last meeting, didn't we?

The coast of Devon and the English Channel did their best to remind me of Italy and the Mediterranean. As the sun set it was really perfect and inland of course it was more lovely than anything ever seen outside this island. She's a dirty careless old Bitch, like a raving beauty who's weary of her lovers, only takes the trouble to wash and make up about three times a year. And the lovers who've been very naturally faithless to her during her months of sluttishness feel contrite that their affections have wondered from their first and exquisite and true love.

How's my Hugo, tell him I'm not at all sure I haven't got a bit of tooth trouble too. Thursday July 29th Goodwood Cup Day, d'you remember Epigram, four years ago, we'll be there again my love, backing all the good things, falling up the stairs, watching the breeze from the sea blow the summer dresses tight against the bodies of the little lovelies, popping in and out of the Champagne Bar, enormously happy and tremendously in love. Nothing can stop it and it shall come again just as certainly as I shall. (Been without it for ten days so I'm bragging a bit.) See you on Wednesday my love, have a nice weekend, Always and always my love to you, Tam.

Tam to Margaret Sidmouth, midnight, 1 August 1942

Oh dear,

'A man is a worriesome thing,
Who leaves you to sing
The blues in the night.
My momma done told me. . .'

My wireless has just been transporting me back to Halfway Cottage. Playing Rummy with you for stakes you never intended to pay, except the lovely evening you tied me up. I believe I'm only realising in retrospect what exquisite happiness I had every hour we were there. Except at about three or four early in the morning of February 20th.[1]

Charming evening last night. Went over to the Marines at 7.30 to dine to discover they'd forgotten, dined early and gone to an E.N.S.A.[2] show. No word of apology today which in their own poverty of expression they would, no doubt, describe as a 'Bad Show' and I with my command of invective would term fucking discourteous, ill-mannered and unpardonable effrontery.

Goodnight and God bless till Wednesday,
Always and always, Tam

1. The time of Hugo's birth.
2. Entertainments National Service Association, popularly called Every Night Something Awful.

Tam to Margaret Sidmouth, Saturday 8 August 1942

Oh my Darling,

What a dreary world it is here today without you. A thick mist envelopes everything. It really is so thick that I found myself contemplating deserting for a day or two, no one would ever discover one's absence.

I wonder if after the War we shall be able to say, well, we managed, we ate and drank and we smoked, we paid a few bills, Hugo was born in comfort and the girls kept at school, we had parties and plenty of fires and weekends together, we had doctors when we were ill and new clothes sometimes. I wonder when we say that we shall feel enormously proud or whether we shall just feel so tired and bored and disappointed at the waste of time, and sickened and sorrowful at the waste of life – what the hell does it matter anyway.

The rain is sweeping across the little tin huts making a hullabaloo against them. It's lonely and desolate and I've been insane enough to order two books from *The Times* both dealing with the miseries and brutalities that have descended on Europe during the last three years.

Hey diddle diddle the cat and the fiddle the Lieutenant jumped over the cliff. Must listen to the news now and have a drink. Hugo will be having his bottle. My love to you all my darling, it was lovely being with you,
Always and always, Tam

Tam to Margaret Sidmouth, Sunday evening, 9 August 1942

My Darling,

This morning I was in the office and heard a 'plane making rather ugly and ominous noises, went out and saw that it was smoking. I watched him crash land it in a tiny field about a mile away. I was there about ten minutes later, it was a Hurricane and burning like hell. The Sergeant Pilot was alright and as cool and collected as you please. The engine had seized. Considering it was a Sunday morning the fire engines were there very quickly and a motley rabble of Home Guard, Firemen, Police and little boys put the fire out. The Sergeant Pilot picked up his parachute harness, told us there were a couple of 250 lbs in the 'plane but assured us with a friendly smile that they wouldn't go off (nothing round here seems intended to explode) and wandered off to the Police Station. The contrast of his lack of concern and the excitement of the locals was really funny – he seemed amused by it too.

I'm glad they've locked up that little weasel Ghandi.[1] Now he'll fast I suppose. But OH Dear I wish we could have some better news from Russia. I suppose Churchill and Joe are arguing the toss through a haze of brandy and the Second Front is discussed over the third bottle.[2] And now we see carried on to another age that imbecile and most loathsome query 'What did you do in the War Mummy' à propos of Firewatching. If Hugo ever makes such an enquiry I shall swipe him across the head with a great lump of iron. But how embarrassing to have to answer, 'I sat on my bottom on the edge of a cliff in Devon, my son, in charge of a small detachment of men and the Canteen money.'

Goodnight my love,
Always and always,
Tam

1. Under Ghandi's influence, on 9 August 1942 the All-India Congress passed a 'Quit India' Resolution which was to have been followed by a campaign of civil disobedience, but Ghandi and the other leaders were imprisoned. The British government was worried about the effect their action might have on the defence of India and on war production.
2. On 13 August 1942 Churchill flew secretly to Moscow for four days of talks with Joseph Stalin.

Tam to Margaret Sidmouth, Tuesday 11 August 1942

Went into Exmouth yesterday, a dreary little place I thought, wandered around and finally went to a cinema. Clark Gable and Loretta Young in *The Call of the Wild*, must have been made at least ten years ago, not bad. It was odd to sit in Charlie Eaton's[1] battle dress in the darkness of that little flea pit and suddenly remember that I'd met Gable. After you've meandered round a strange town in which you know nobody, you begin to think you've never known anybody, anywhere, ever. I began to feel nearer to the creatures on the screen, whom I could claim as acquaintances, than I did to the W.A.A.F. who sat next to me and whose proximity was emphasised by a strong smell of sweat.

I'm due for forty eight hours on Saturday Fortnight. I wish we were at Newmarket. No I don't, I wish we were lying in the sun somewhere looking after Hugo for the afternoon while Nannie was taken out in a glass-bottomed boat to see the coloured fish.

Always my darling, Tam

1. Charles Eaton, friend of Tam and Margaret's, living at Dorney.

Tam to Margaret Sidmouth, Wednesday 12 August 1942

My Darling,

Still blowing up on my hill. If I'm here in the winter I shall fasten myself to the ground, but if I'm here in the winter I'll be raving mad anyway. Dear God it's boring.

A letter from you this afternoon, thank you for writing so often my darling, your letters are an enormous comfort. I love you so much my sweet and each day apart seems like a week, a week of

complete waste of time. But that's the price that happy people in love with each other have to pay. It's all perfect when they're together, but when they're separated the light goes out of life. Life just doesn't continue until they meet again. The six o'clock blues coming up. August the 12th doesn't mean 5/- for a little brown bird usually a year old any more does it? Oysters and grouse and cobnuts, Krug '28, Kummel and coffee. I've just been reading an account of the Finnish War and am now very muddled. It is Russia we're rooting for this time isn't it? I wonder which is worse, to keep sane in a world gone mad or go mad in a world still sane. Maybe I'll let you know sometime.
Forever and ever, Tam

Tam to Margaret Sidmouth, Friday 14 August 1942

My Darling,

This is my busy day, Pay Parade at 4.30 which takes a good forty minutes. A thick grey mist this morning, everything damp, clothes, cigarettes, and the sugar lumps itself and envelopes stick themselves up.

Nowadays one continually reads of 'The greatest battle the world has ever seen is raging etc etc.' 'Enormous casualties', and people forget that on July 1st 1916 the British Army sustained 60,000 casualties in one day, which is considered now a large figure for a months' fighting. But the Generals of this War were Company Commanders in the last War, they saw their men and their subalterns slaughtered worthlessly, life was chucked away without any gain, and that stuck. In the English mind it stuck, in the German it was forgotten. Ever since this War started the Higher Ups have tried to conduct it with the minimum of senseless casualties. During training it was always being impressed upon us that if we were killed it would not be in the same needless way the chaps were killed in the last War. They would never forget the horror of seeing men strung up on the wire while enemy machine guns picked them off like bottles at a fair. What's the result? Surrenders, withdrawals, errors. No one should blame a general because his conscience seizes him and his humanity suddenly screams in his head 'I'm killing people stupidly' and he closes the battle. 'He lost his nerve' they say, but they haven't the sense to see that he didn't lose it in the Western Desert in 1942 but at the battle of the Somme in 1916. It all comes under the heading of 'C'est la guerre' and so I suppose does the bombing of Seaton at 7 o'clock the evening before last where they killed an old woman of 91, and of Truro last week where they hit the Infirmary. I swear to you I'd sooner have the toothache and think of that than to think of what's going on in the world today. It's being alone and having nothing to do. At Denham one forgot the War. I was talking to Sgt. Pollard the other evening. 'You know our motto?' he said. 'You know wot her means?' 'Yes,' I said. 'Forever Faithful'. 'No Sor. You'm wrong Sor – we've got a new one now, it's Fuck you Jack, I'm fine'.

Has Hugo reached the photogenic stage yet? I mean is anyone going to be able to produce a picture which, in years to come, will neither fill him with disgust nor us with remorse? If so let's get someone down on my next leave and have the well-known group, Mum, Dad, the Brat and the Dogs. Suitable for Grand Pianos and insertion in the Tatler.

Take care of yourself my darling, my love to them all and thank you for writing,

For always and always, Tam

My love and I we used to go
Down Bond St for a stroll.
We sauntered slowly passed the shops
Leisurely towards our goal
Which was generally the Berkeley
For a pint of Monopole,
And on the way we used to stop
And buy a buttonhole.

But that was all sometime ago,
Two summers and a spring,
Alas! My red carnation's gone,
You cannot wear the thing
Pinned into the uniform
Of His Majesty the King.

My love and I will wait awhile
To buy a buttonhole
And once again look in the shops
Of Bond St as we stroll.
But it's very clearly understood
The Berkeley's still our goal
And Peace Aims certainly include
A pint of Monopole.

Tam to Margaret Sidmouth, Sunday morning, 16 August 1942

A month since I saw Hugo. I wonder so often what the world will be like for him. I think it will be a better world, but not so nice, and yet I don't know. There wasn't anything particularly nice about the thirties, and the twenties were thought to be definitely nasty. I'm certain I shall find myself boring him dreadfully with remarks like 'They can't cook here like they used to' or 'Yes, but you should have seen so and so' and 'Oh it was lovely when your mother and I came here first, now they've spoilt it'. All parents do, I suppose. It bestows an immense glamour on the years just before your own experience and memory began. I've always thought the Edwardian days must have been infinitely wonderful, or is it because that wonderful world came tumbling down in 1914?

God I'm sick of people bleating about the next 80 days, the next 60 days. The Sunday Papers are full of '20 days have now passed' etc. It all sounds like some ghastly period of quarantine and it makes it appear twice as long saying it in days. 'Forty days and forty nights' always sounds a hell of a lot longer than six weeks.
God bless you my precious, my love to you for always. Love to the Grandmothers and my Hugo.
Tam

Tam to Margaret Sidmouth, Wednesday 19 August 1942

Pouring with rain and a heavy sea mist and one's clothes feel like the inside of a sponge bag. Blast, I missed you again last night, by five minutes. I'd been having dinner, two roast chickens appeared, one I regarded as quite extraordinary and for two I think there should be a new collective noun invented. A sufficiency of Hens.

Tell me if you hear why Auckinleck is out now.[1] Our Generals seem to come and go as quickly as general servants. They'll have to start a system of references, make up their minds and at last admit to the Terrified Public that at last Mr Churchill is 'Settled'. I wonder what's going on in Dieppe,[2] there was a hell of a lot of noise in the Channel last night and the night before I saw stuff being dropped across the mouth of the river, Teignmouth I imagine, within a few seconds the all clear went. Really it's very amateur after all the practice they must have had.

I've been made an Hon. Member of the Exmouth Club so might get some Bridge. I believe there's an actor called Gerald Lawrence in Exmouth I used to play with at the Green Room Club. He got the worst notice from St John Ervine[3] I've ever read: 'Mr Gerald Lawrence played the part of Tosca's lover as though he'd just drunk a pint of Brilliantine.'

We had the most ghastly E.N.S.A. show here yesterday. I've sent in a stinking report urging that every safeguard should be taken to ensure against the danger of American troops being subjected to such entertainment. I really don't know what they'd do. Tanks taken to Dieppe! Sounds rather like a final dress rehearsal doesn't it? And what about Churchill's funny hats – He looked like some old Bartender in Tia Juana. See you soon my lovely Margaret. I have to keep saying 'See you soon' otherwise I get low. My love to everyone and to you my Darling forever and ever, Tam.

1. General Auckinleck was replaced by General Alexander as Churchill wanted somebody more overtly aggressive to take over the leadership of the North Africa Campaign.
2. Combined Canadian and British raid on Dieppe, planned as a fore-runner to D-Day.
3. St John Ervine was a playwright, author of *The First Mrs Frazer* and sometime Drama Critic of the *Observer*.

Tam to Margaret — Sidmouth, Friday 21 August 1942

Hunting for some paper I came across my old notes from Officer Cadet Training, December 1939. They included pages on the formation of a French Infantry Division and a lecture on Trench Warfare. I felt that the War had been in progress for a long time more acutely than ever before. Dear God, what a lot of red tape has flowed from the desks of Whitehall since those days. And now one's keeness is blunted and instead of that comforting feeling that one had, at any rate, lost no time in getting busy, now one feels that all one does is so futile, so utterly, miserably, hopelessly futile. Pouring with rain and mist and the drip drip drip on the tin roofs. I found this pearl of great price nestling in the Battery Orders this morning. Subject: Breakfast Cereal.

'It is desirable that rat bait (poisoned oatmeal) should not be served in lieu of porridge (oatmeal)'

I wonder was the Dieppe raid merely a raid or was it something else that was hastily converted into a raid. That's fairly fifth column talk I admit, but through all this second front talk one is haunted by the fear that we shall be kicked into the sea for the fifth or the sixth time.

Longing to see you my precious one. Hullo to Hugo and my love to the Grannies.

Forever my darling, Tam

Tam to Margaret Sidmouth, Friday 28 August 1942

Isn't it sickening my darling, it's the most perfect day, Summer as it was meant to be, sunny and balmy with a dainty little breeze and a haze on the Channel. But all this peace was sharply interrupted at about 10.45. There's been a lot of noise coming from the sea since quite early and then suddenly that well-remembered screaming and gun-fire and roaring. There were three planes, two Spitfires and a Hun. One Spitfire was in trouble and so was the Hun and the other Spitfire was going faster than anything I've ever seen and behaving like a dog with sheep. He seemed to be chasing the Hun straight out to sea and I noticed they were heading slap over Exmouth. In a second or so the Hun crashed straight into the haze and the sea. The one o'clock news said, 'This morning a raider was shot down in the sea off the South West Coast.' And so, we all thought, was the Spitfire. Pollard highly excited – 'Look at 'ee, look at 'ee, can you see'er Sor, can you see 'er?'

The other Spitfire circled and a few minutes later we saw motor boats tearing out of the mouth of the Exe. I wonder if old Pollard's father who's never been in a train and can't read and is eighty-five looked up from his chickens to behold this battle of a dozen seconds covering, in that time, practically the entire boundaries of his whole world.

The news is working up to the breathless stage again. September always has something for us. God if the Russian plan is really to re-take Smolensk, and they do; and Stalingrad holds, and the Caucusus engulf and bury their attackers. They've got a cause. They're not only fighting for their own land and to revenge the blood of their people and to fling the Germans out of the country, they're fighting madly, blindly for their faith in their political system. Is anyone in England satisfied that our Government is worth dying for?

My Darling it was wonderful having you here and the world seems empty today.

Always my Darling, Tam

Tam to Margaret Sidmouth, Sunday 30 August 1942

The rain it raineth every day, drip drip drip on the bicycle pump. Thank you for your letter my Darling. There's good news from all quarters. The Solomons (they always sound like Tailors, not Islands), Stalingrad holding, the Moscow-Kalenin fronts pushing on, more big raids. As soon as there's a glimmer of hope I do my Celandine act and feel the War is won and the Army done with. The only soldiers I ever wish to see again will be either at Olympia, the Aldershot Tattoo, or in the Bandstand at Ascot. I must go and watch my gang making a path. I sent them blackberrying yesterday. Friday evening when I went to Exeter I wore my side cap. Pollard saw me just as I was leaving. 'Oh – Oh!' Quite startled, then 'Sooner 'ave yew in your peak cap Sor.' God he makes me laugh. My love to you all my darlings, how I love you. Tam

Tam to Margaret

Sidmouth, Monday morning, 31 August 1942

Oh my Darling,

A week today and I shall be with you. It's extraordinary how I look on Halfway Cottage as home. I know nothing in it's ours, nothing reflects us, it's just a temporary Wartime refuge but somehow it is Home. It's a hell of a time since either of us had one, I suppose that's why. I never felt Ashley Place was mine and the Albany was only 5 degrees more comfortable than this inner tube I'm living in now. We'll have a fire, won't we? It's as damp as the inside of a sponge bag again today, thick mist, I shall have to take Kurschen Salts if I'm here in the winter otherwise I'll seize up with rheumatism.

I was appalled at the Air Ministry's announcement yesterday that during the last twelve months we had achieved only 40% of our long term Bombing Programme. What does Churchill do now? I'm certain bombing was going to be his get out for the Second Front and if our Bombing is as weak as that, what explanation is he going to give this country, let alone Russia, in three months time when we have failed to open up a Second Front? I think he'll go. I was thinking yesterday, first we had Baldwin's pipe – British, stupid, insular, apparently honest. Then the Umbrella – caution, let's be on the safe side but I think this may turn out alright, and now the Cigar – arrogant, power-loving, swaggering cock of the weak.

I've started a short story. A miserable, horrible tale. I'm trying to tell it through the medium of Army Forms – personal sorrows, problems and even sudden tragedies seem so extra dreadful when they're set down in block capitals on an Army Form. Crude, blunt, no sympathy, no heart. If I finish it by the end of the week I'll bring it up. Something to do anyway. I remember we had a chap at Bexhill whose mother was killed in the Blitz. He was sent home at once of course, money given, train warrant and a truck to the station, but the pro rata form had to be completed. 'Sir I have the honour to apply for compassionate leave, my reason being etc etc, hoping this will meet with your kind approval I am your obedient servant etc etc.' Well, there's something simply catastrophic about that. There's a million times more drama in that than a red-eyed soldier saying brokenly and wildly 'I've got to get home Sir my Mum's been 'it and she's dying Sir, I've got to get home.' Don't you agree? But my tale is so heartbreaking that after three enormous whiskies last night I was still sobbing quietly. Have I no humour? Why is it my mind always goes morbid on me? Maybe it's the Welsh influence.

All my love beloved, Tam

Margaret to Tam Halfway Cottage, Friday (undated) 1942

My Beloved,

How disappointing. I can't bear to think that you may not come after all. I shall go ahead with my plans for you just the same anyway, of *course* you must have some 'leave' before you go into hospital and we will stay in London for one night.

Well I thoroughly enjoyed *Secret Mission* darling, really much better than *The Day will Dawn* and except for Michael Wilding[1] being hopelessly miscast and James Mason's impression of a Maori Jewish Frenchman who was extremely sorry for himself, and Miss Lehmann's[2] *dead*pan acting (?) it was much better and far less disjointed. You were really excellent and looked grand I thought, all very light and not at all heroish, for my God what a Flash Gordon you could have been. Saw what you meant about the end. Miss L could have, if she'd been an actress, made everyone leave the theatre in floods of tears. More about it all when I see you.

How is your story, is it finished? If so bring it up for me to read please.

Shall express this from Windsor for you darling and pop in a fiver.

How I'm longing to see you my love. God bless you always and always,

Your own, M.

I *do* love you.

1. Michael Wilding (1912–79), actor, at one time married to Elizabeth Taylor.
2. Beatrix Lehmann (1903–79), actress.

Tam to Margaret

Cambridge Hospital, Aldershot,
Friday 18 September 1942

My Darling,

I finally got back this evening but in a very bad temper. Two bottles, my cigars, my fruit, my stick and that curious gypsy bundle took some considerable controlling. Things fell out all over the station at Ascot, where I had to wait for an hour so I left them in a heap where they lay and went over to the pub. There was a wonderfully refined little woman there, slightly boosey. I was busy reading my paper and only caught one or two remarks: 'During Jimmy's leave I must have had a hundred Guinesses' and 'What's that he's got growing out of his forehead dear?'

I wonder how my Prudie is getting on today?[1] I don't believe she'll mind a bit and she's got Loo. My first day of course is an absolute beacon of misery and terror which I can still remember as vividly as anything in my life.

I'm being moved down into a ward for two this evening, no wireless. If I said I wanted to hear the news it would be useless. They don't even stop talking when it's being read.

My love to Hugo and to your darling self. God Bless.

Always and always, Tam

P.S. Twice this morning I've been asked by these female impersonators if it 'really is fixed for you tomorrow?' Sounds fishy and how the hell should I know anyway. Maybe I'll see you at the Windsor races yet!

1. Prue's first day at Cheltenham Ladies' College.

Tam to Margaret

Cambridge Hospital, Sunday morning,
21 September 1942

Thank you for telephoning my darling. Everything gone according to plan. Went down to the theatre about 9.30 yesterday morning and at 11.30 in this new ward, with a filthy taste and very pissy. Slept and dozed most of the day. Saw the Doctor who told me the cartilage was badly torn, so it's comforting to know it would never have got right.

Had a somewhat uncomfortable night and slept little. Morphia tonight so shall be OK, but so far the pain has certainly not come up to all the stories everyone delighted in telling me.

Will you come over on Wednesday, my darling, I shall want some pyjamas. How's my Hugo. Love to you all. Always and always, Tam

Tam to Margaret Cambridge Hospital, 24 September 1942

Darling,

Thank you for coming over yesterday, it must be a hell of a toil and thank you my pretty for lugging over the radio, which makes a big difference. You are sweet to me aren't you? And I love you more and more and in so many ways, so kind you are and so sweet and such fun and so lovely. Though at the moment I detect a certain austerity in hats, those little felt numbers, they're buggers, and the result of your living in the English country where hats are worn to keep off the wind and rain. There was a natural reaction to this when you got that little floozie bluezie thing, which of course was a bugger too. I think I'm probably better at hats than you.

It looks a simply lovely morning. I wish we could walk somewhere, everything we do together now seems so vivid and important, no I don't mean that. I mean, maybe, that we find ourselves in such funny places, and so often saying goodbye and so often saying Hello that the present seems sometimes already a memory. D'you follow me?

Share all of my love with Hugo. I love you so very much. God bless you darling, Tam

Tam to Margaret Cambridge Hospital, Wednesday evening, 1 October 1942

Oh my Dear Girl,

I cannot help writing to you this very instant to record the exquisite feelings I have. A bath, a Tom, a Whisky and a cigarette. OH BOY OH BOY I feel as bien soigné and hotsy totsy as any little Park Avenue floozie. True some horrible meal will soon appear and I shall feel normal once again but at the moment it is really something.

Oh Darling, I drink to you, to your two most lovely lips, to your eyes, to that so very perfect nose, to that peerless skin and to the wondrous bones beneath. To all the happiness we've shared and all the happiness you've given and to all the moments in the future when I shall be thankful for your sweetness and your kindness and grateful for the likeness to you that I see in Hugo. I love you very dearly. . .

Well it was time something interrupted that mood of ecstacy, but I certainly hadn't counted on 'Chinese Noodles' – Dear God in Heaven! Reinforced rubber hosing sprinkled with Army issue soap, heated and allowed to congeal. Served with a smile on a stone cold plate. They ought to be fucking well flogged these bloody cooks. Period of digestion up to ninety six hours. It's now 6.40 and not another morsel till 8.30 tomorrow morning. I shall have a couple of tomatoes and some walnuts around midnight. Now I'm going to do my exercises. Goodnight Beloved – maybe one of the reasons my writing is so poor is on account of I'm in bed.

Good morning my darling. What a lovely-looking morning. I say this school is awful, the casualties are over forty now. God it's awful isn't it? I think the eldest was only about eleven. It gives one's heart a sort of cramp. I can read about men in open boats for forty days and hostages being shot and women living in holes in the sand alright now, but little boys being killed in a Sussex village. . .

I didn't like that bit about Dunkirk and Dieppe being great British victories, compared to which, of course, our conquests seem trivial! That made me quite embarrassed. The man in the next bed has just had a rubber tube shoved down his throat into his stomach – horrible noise. 'What's the matter with you, I had that for supper, put some mustard on it.' A screen was quickly brought and I got a dirty look. Love to you all,
Tam

Margaret to Tam Halfway Cottage, 30 December 1942

Beloved,

I've just heard 'I'll be seeing you' on the radio and for no reason I suddenly remembered my birthday 2 years ago, when you got me pissy and then got angry because I could not see my way down the hill in Windsor and I lost my mink hat. You borrowed a torch from a soldier to look for it, found it and tipped him 2/6 before you realised he was a captain. Golly how we laughed then. Remember? Oh I love being with you my Tamèd.

Had a letter from you this morning dated 23rd. I thought a little gritty about my letters. You said you knew I wrote them in a hurry. Some of them, yes, others no. I don't hurry because I don't *like* writing them, it's usually because I have so much to say to you that it comes tumbling out. I want to write to you as I talk. I love to try and tell you everything that goes on. Please don't write a gritty letter again because I mean well and I love you so much.

You said nothing about the Hun offensive. Oh golly I hope it does not slow the end too much. I'm much more cheerful about it now that the R.A.F. are back on the job. Bloody awful Hitler weather. It is still terribly cold here, but clear skies and a pale trickle of sunlight to thaw out the world.

I'd adore to see Prue's anthology. What a lovely record of the sort of girl she is. You must be proud.

I hear Hugo waking now I think, so I'll go and get him. Be good, take care of yourself, continue to love me in spite of all. I love you now and always and always,
Your own M.

Tam to Margaret Northwood, Middlesex, 30 December 1942

My Darling,

I wrote to you a week or so ago, but as I thought we'd probably have a chance to talk I didn't send it, which is a pity now for it might have saved us Monday night.

We're going through something now, that we've really been wonderfully lucky not to have had to face during the last three and a half years. I mean that the War is making us unhappy. Until now we've hardly been separated and although I was hating the Army and you were living in snow and discomfort and we were broke and had trouble with landlords, we were happy. Then there were the wonderful times before and after you had Hugo. And now the War is well in its fourth year and we're not finding it as easy to take as we did a couple of years ago. Nanny is a worry, the housework is gradually making you feel you're a drudge, Ruby[1] not being well hasn't helped, you're worried about having another baby too soon after Hugo, and it's Winter. Well, if your mind works anything like mine you think like this: I mustn't grumble but Oh Dear God I'm fed up, I wonder if anyone, even Tam, realises just how fed up I am. I shall see him soon, perhaps he'll solve a problem or two and anyway I can talk to him, that'll be something.

Meanwhile in the cold loneliness of Northwood I'm thinking when can I get home again? How soon shall I see Margaret? Dear God I'm fed up. I mustn't grumble when I go home, all the same I wonder if she realises just how much I loathe the Army. I wonder if she or anyone else realises that these are such vitally important and precious years for me and I'm missing them and if the War goes on much longer I shall only be fit to play Family Solicitors and Kindly Fathers.

Here, let me add, that through one thing or another, not being well, being tired, being tight, being separated, we've practically lived without beising, and remember there is an enormous comfort to be got out of beising. It wasn't just thought of to make babies and to have moments of ecstacy in their making. Well, now we've denied ourselves that. My fault more than yours. Now, lets remember that you've not been well and that I've not been well, that we've had no holiday, no sun or privacy for literally years. And then I arrive, tired, at your busiest moment of the the day while you're getting the dinner. I rush for the Whisky and the longing for each other that's helped us through the week, the waiting for the understanding and comfort we've looked forward to ends in disappointment. We both become convinced that the other is only conscious of his or her own troubles and doesn't give a hoot in hell about the other. Oh my Darling, my darling, that isn't true. But that's how it sometimes seems and although I blame myself for most of it I think that in a lesser degree it's your fault too. It's a testing time and if we get through it we'll be happier later on, but if we boob and take it badly it'll make us lose faith in each another. I love you more than I ever did, I know most surely than I ever did my happiness is entirely centred in you and Hugo. You'll get this on New Year's Day and so you'll know what my resolution is. A Happy New Year, it'll be exciting I think, and maybe happy in the Autumn.

That's all, except to say how miserable my part in all this has made me. It's only a passing boob that's finished now, and God wot we can find excuses in plenty for not being our own real selves. Give my love and Happy 1943 to everyone. Always and always my Darling, Tam

1. Ruby was Margaret's mother and lived with her for the duration of the war.

1943

Crowded in my solitude,
This, I proffer, Sirs
To the nouns of multitude:
A mess of Officers.

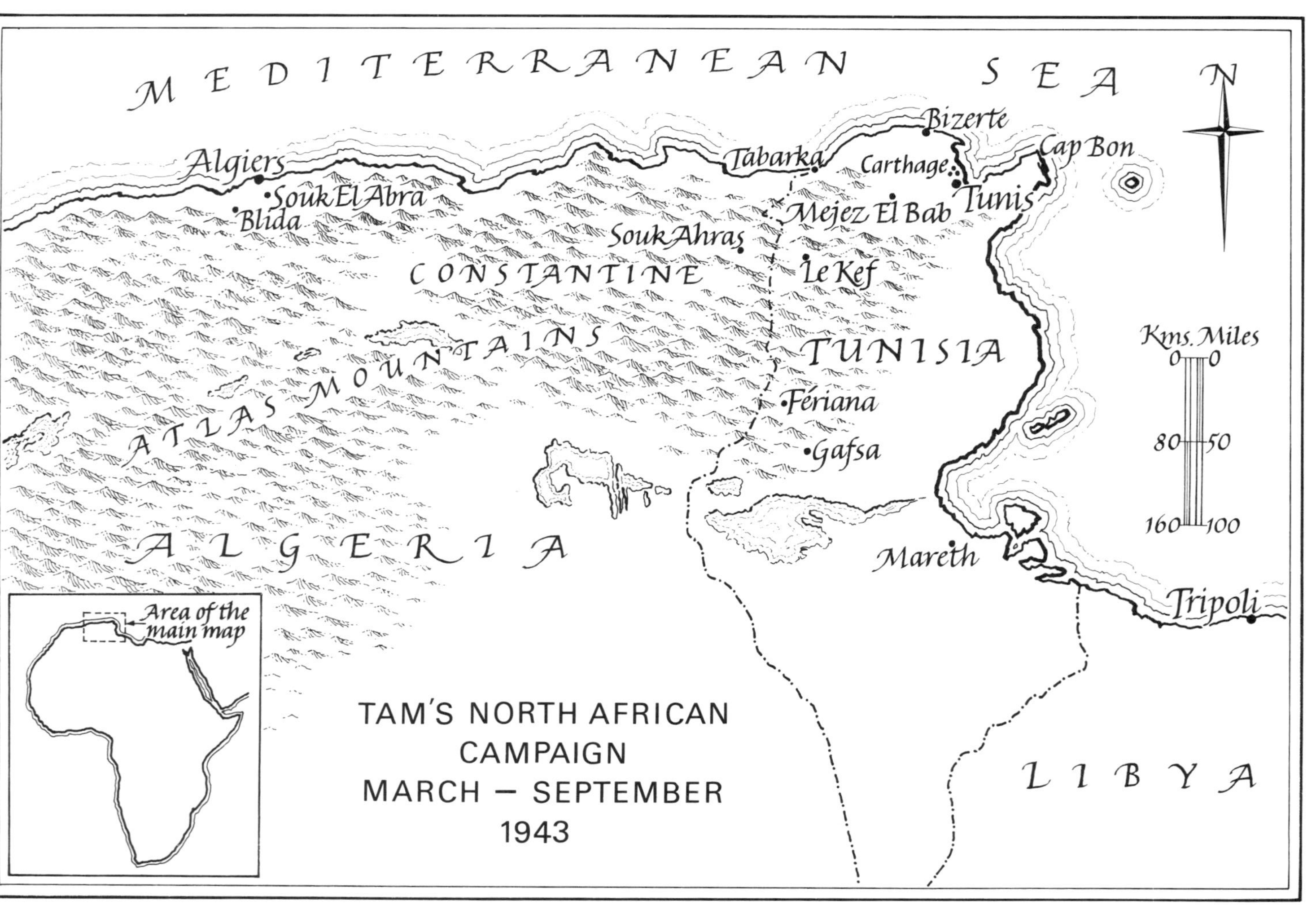
MEDITERRANEAN SEA
N
Algiers
Souk El Abra
Blida
Tabarka
Bizerte
Carthage
Tunis
Cap Bon
Mejez El Bab
Souk Ahras
Le Kef
CONSTANTINE
ATLAS MOUNTAINS
TUNISIA
Fériana
Gafsa
Mareth
Tripoli
Kms. Miles
0 0
80 50
160 100
ALGERIA
LIBYA
Area of the main map
TAM'S NORTH AFRICAN
CAMPAIGN
MARCH – SEPTEMBER
1943

At last Tam was about to see service abroad. He was posted to Tunisia as part of the North Africa Campaign, where he served in 'K' Squadron of Phantom, a regiment that specialized in intelligence gathering and had units based wherever there was fighting. He probably had to pull strings in order to be transferred.

Tam to Margaret 19 February 1943

Well My Darling,

You were simply splendid – I kept thinking how strange that Shakespeare's wisdom should have so far deserted him as to make him write anything so utterly incorrect as 'Parting is such sweet sorrow' – I suppose he thought of the last line of the couplet first – 'That I would say goodnight till it be morrow'. Which is sense. But for sheer concentrated hideous anguish I think yesterday achieved a new high. And I'm glad that we had that minute or two when we stopped behaving like a couple of characters in a Coward play, and emotion took over. To hell with people with feelings so atrophied and hearts so little that to control them is a simple matter. Tears are to be shed – not to trickle backwards to make one more unhappy. And by God how good to think that the very, very worst moment of all is behind us – we've said goodbye, and now the next words are 'Hello again'.

I hope Hugo has assumed his new role of only man of the family with good heart.

Quite an elegant ship,[1] though a little crowded! I found myself wandering round in the well-remembered way and old instincts, like complaining about my cabin, fixing a good table, ordering a bottle, and finding a strategic place from which to check the market, had to be rapidly overcome. Even now I feel I should be looking out for the Smoking Room Steward to put my name down for the sweep.

I've a top bunk with Edward Oliver,[2] who has been unpacking and perspiring for seven hours underneath me, as well as eighteen other subaltern officers in the cabin which is going to seem uncomfortably like the men's crowd room at Denham[3] I fancy.

Today is Hugo's birthday. I wonder if you'll be remembering the lines from *Dierdre* I read to you a year ago while we were waiting for him. 'And I shall remember nothing but that old vehement, bewildering kiss.'[4] God bless him and you my darling, thank you for giving him to me and for all the fun and happiness, and the lovely future round the bend. Shaving and dressing this morning

was really something. No chorus on a first night ever got into more of a shambles. I love you my beloved and by now you know I always shall.
Tam

1. Tam sailed on the SS *Buissevain*.
2. Edward Oliver served with Tam in Phantom.
3. The room where the film extras waited at Denham Studios.
4. Tam is misquoting from *Dierdre*, a play by W.B. Yeats: 'And I know nothing but this body, Nothing but that old vehement bewildering kiss.' Yeats dedicated the play to Mrs Patrick Campbell, the actress who created the title role. Mrs Pat, as she was known, was a great friend of Tam's and godmother to his daughter Loo.

Tam to Margaret

Docked on the Clyde at Glasgow
waiting to sail for North Africa
Sunday 21 February 1943

There is still another post, so another letter to my love. The name of this ever so chic stationery is Marina and I purchased it at the shop where they also sell blotting pads made in wood from Batavia, contraceptives and Australian opals, Mackintoshes toffee and Owbridges Lung Tonic. I behaved rather like you at the Vicarage Sale. We jockeyed about yesterday rather like the start of the Hunt Cup.

There were twenty seven people – including servants – in our Cabin de Luxe this morning, which is about the size of the dining room at home. However I have discovered a little place with a basin near the lounge on the Boat Deck with the word Dames over the door and such is the chivalry of Englishmen that even on a troop ship the word means something, and it is invariably empty. The piano is still the main agony – we had 'In a Monastery Garden' at 8.15 this morning. How sorry I am that I ever said an unkind word about the Palmers Arms, in my nostalgia it seems the very Elysium of alcohol. (How odd that I should have difficulty spelling that word!)

Tony's[1] training programme has been carried through today in the face of terrific difficulties. The first period was interrupted by the Captain's ship inspection. P.T. was cancelled because the decks were being washed – then during the next period there was suddenly a boat drill – a mad rush to lock up the code books and grab a life belt. Imagine all seven classes being conducted simultaneously by various officers in an extremely confined space somewhere where any normal ship has its engines. I look forward, but only out of sheer curiosity, to the same scene in even a moderate sea.

Write again soon, God bless and all my love to you and a manly kiss for my boy,
Tam

1. Major J.A. Warre MC, Tam's commanding officer.

Margaret to Tam Halfway Cottage, 22 February 1943

My own Beloved,

Here I am back in Halfway Cottage with Hugo. TaTa for now you said in your wire. I wonder how long it will be. It has been a wonderful and happy year here, but now that you are not here, I don't really want to stay. Too many memories to live with. Johnny took me to The Peroquet on Thursday the 18th and poured brandy into me. Strange, but nothing happened at all, nerves very tightly gripped or something, but I left completely sober, rang Nanny and Hugo and to bed quite early at The Connaught. Then to the studio early next morning for hair tests. Saw Larry[1] and gave him your address. He sent his love.

Saturday 20th

Funny last night at midnight I could not get you out of my mind. Wonder if you were with me darling. I felt very close and yet so lonely. My beloved I love you so terribly, for ever and ever.

Hugo has had a wonderful birthday, he came in to wake me this morning and got his presents. A duck on wheels from you and me and of course your telegram. He put his best suit on for tea – just Nanny and me. We will have a party for him on March 6th and drink you a toast darling, in orange juice! He was thinking of you at 6 o'clock tonight. I know, for he sat and looked so dreamy and serious when I told him to think of Dada.

Darling the moon is full again, is it the 42nd or the 43rd? I wonder how many moons it will be until we are together again. This letter is only a short one. Let me know how long it takes to get to you my love as I'm going to try various ways and means to see which is quickest. You are always in my thoughts my love and take care of yourself remember. I'm loving you every moment of the day.
Always and always, your M.

1. Laurence Olivier (1907–89), actor. He was a friend of Tam's and gave the address at his memorial service in 1969.

Tam to Margaret 24 February 1943

Well My Darling,

We finally sailed about midnight on Wednesday. By that time, as you might imagine, one was becoming very bored with the scenery. Yesterday was a bad day, one of those swells which look harmless but make the ship do everything except 'go bang'. I spent the day fairly comfortably, mostly watching the convoy. The biggest thrill of the war. It's real Dogs of War stuff and the news reels give one no idea of it. Very very exciting and I felt that maybe though there won't forever be a girl called Gertie Lawrence[1], There'll always be an England. However one's moments of national pride were continually interrupted by nausea and dodging what the less imaginative at first presumed was spray. Most people retired, only old pissers like Springett,[2] Tony and myself remaining.

I've found myself what at the moment looks like a good servant – he's done my washing today which is fortunate for one now sleeps clothed so two sets of things are needed, those that smell for the privacy of the bunk, those that don't for the day time. There are a score of cases of the dear stuff aboard at 6 /- a bottle – but under lock and key. But cigarettes are 1/8 for fifty and there's nothing but butter served so far. If you can divide two thousand seven hundred by twenty three – take away two because they're out of order – you will arrive at the number of lavatories per man. Enos has to be timed very carefully.

Remarks which amused – 'No Hugh Williams is not on board, it's Leslie Banks'[3] and 'I don't mind what you wear for Boat Drill, but if it's a real torpedo we'll wear Berets.'

During my duty watch on the bridge – midnight to four and quite the most boring thing I've done since guarding Staines Bridge – the ship in front took a sharp left turn and I inquired why. 'Somebody's gone to sleep, be alright in a minute.'

The last couple of days I've realised what an appalling time this bloody war has been on. Three and a half years ago last night since we walked out of the Stage Door of the Queens Theatre and into the Queen's Westminsters.[4]

It's time to join the queue for the shop – more later my beloved. I wonder how soon it will be before we lean over the rail of a ship together and watch the phosphorous and the stars. Haven't had a drink for two days. D'you follow my train of thought? In my mind's eye there was a bottle cooling in a bucket while I was making outrageous love to you on the deck. T.T.F.N. Which looks so like a code I'd better translate it for the censor. Ta ta for now my darling.

A ship is always a magnificent ground for rumours – 'So and so's a card cheat', 'We're not touching at Naples because of the Small Pox' – I shall say I've seen a seal and it's getting colder, and I bet you by midday tomorrow someone will say we're headed for Iceland.

To say I miss you is utterly absurd. I am incomplete. I am never quite anywhere for some part of my mind is following your daily round, picturing and imagining how you are and if you're looking lovely or just pretty. There's a tune with the first two or three bars exactly like 'Always and Always' – d'you know the one I mean? Some bugger will whistle it and then my heart goes bang and missing you becomes not just something that goes on all the time, but like a great blow with a lump of lead in the middle of the chest. God bless you always,
Tam

1. Gertrude Lawrence (1898–1952), musical comedy actress, she often partnered Noël Coward.
2. Captain S.S. Demetriadi, known as Dick Springett, a friend of Tam's.
3. Leslie Banks (1890–1952), film and stage actor.
4. Tam was appearing at the Queen's Theatre in the West End when he enlisted in the Territorial Army.

Margaret to Tam — Halfway Cottage, 25 February 1943

My own Tamèd

Same old me sitting in the same little chair by the fire, pulling it a little closer and yet closer in a vain endeavour to get warm, although we've had some more lovely days. I always have difficulty in starting my letters to you, for there seems to be so many things to say and it's difficult to know where to begin. Hugo is virtually walking now and very excited about it. Oh I wish you'd been here to see him, he sets off across the room with a fixed expression on his face, then something attracts his attention and of course he loses his balance and then down he goes.

David and Prim[1] are moving into Flaxford, the Clydes house, and Eliza[2] is moving into another little house opposite the Palmers' Arms. She says she wants somewhere permanent and Flaxford is only on a monthly basis and may be wanted at any moment by the owner. Johnny[3] says David says he is not going to make a film, which is good reason to believe he is.

I wonder where you are as I write this, perhaps you have gone to bed by now for it is nearly 10 o'clock, or maybe you've gone out on deck to feel the sea air on your face and hear the sound of the sea as it dashes against the sides of the ship. It must be strange to feel that there might be danger in the sea after all the wonderful gay trips you've made without even thinking of safety. And perhaps you are thinking of Hugo and me.

I did tell you that we are having Hugo's party on your birthday? We shall all be thinking of you darling and hoping that we shall be together next time. Suppose by the time you read this you will have seen your 'Place in the sun'. Ye Gods that we should not be together. Churchill better,[4] Roosevelt ill, news better and I love and miss you every moment of the day.

Always your M.

1. David Niven (1909–83), film star, and his wife Primula.
2. The Clydes lived in Dorney. Tommy served in the Horse Guards and Eliza (Lady Elizabeth) was the daughter of the Seventh Duke of Wellington. Their son Jeremy, born in 1941, was Hugo's best friend.
3. Johnny Hannay.
4. On 17 February Churchill was taken ill with pneumonia.

Margaret to Tam — Halfway Cottage, 27 February 1943

My beloved,

Have been to London for the day, what a really miserable day, my first there since you left and as you know I was beginning to dislike it quite a lot before. Now it really is ghastly and with these lovely sunny days it makes London look so very old and shabby and world and war weary. Rather like I feel when I'm caught in early spring with no new dresses – peace time I mean – As I sat in the buses and tube watching other couples, so seldom attractive, particularly in pairs, I felt the most frightful nostalgia for you and the look of you and the proud swelling in my heart and throat as I look at you and know you are mine.

My ever carefully guarded loneliness here has been a bit invaded by well-wishers since you left. Sort of poor old Maggie mustn't let her get lonely thing. All very kind and sweet but God how I hate it. As I get older there are less and less people I want to be with, so darling at this rate one morning I'll wake up and only want to see you and Hugo ever, so *please* be back by then.

Always and always in my heart and thoughts,

Your M.

Margaret to Tam — Halfway Cottage, 4 March 1943

Tamèd my Tam,

Once again I sit before the fire. I've just had an egg and a glass of milk and I feel very cosy, but I'd give anything in the whole world just for a look at you darling.

Another huge raid on Berlin on Monday. We lost 19, so it must have been big. They came back in a very small way last night, a bit noisy here but no damage in the district. The news in North Africa[1] has cheered me up a lot lately. Maybe it won't be so long eh darling?

Suppose you felt pretty miserable on your way to wherever you went. I lay thinking about you all night, wondering how you felt and hoping you were not going off with a worried heart about your gaggle.

I'll write to you on Sat my darling love to wish you a happy (Ye Gods) birthday. We seem doomed to be apart for your birthday don't we?

Goodnight and God bless you. Hugo and I love you always and always, your M.

1. On 26 February American troops drove the Germans, led by Rommel, out of the mountains of Central Tunisia.

Margaret to Tam — Halfway Cottage, 7 March 1943

My beloved my love,

I light a cigarette, I sit gratefully in front of our fire. The last three days have been hectic so I've saved up my news to write to you now that all is quiet and I have the place to myself.

The very thought of sixteen small people as Hugo's guests has been far worse than any of our Christmas parties. And as it was his first party I was mad keen for it to be a success. The day chosen was lucky, your birthday – or is it? We always seem to be apart. Or perhaps the ones we are not together for don't count, so that shortly we shall be the same age.

All day Friday I borrowed cups and saucers, fireguards, mugs, cooked and cooked and fussed and fumed. Finally went to bed at 4.30 AM. I iced his cake with chocolate and wrote Hugo in marshmallows, then put a small china dog and a candle on top. Not bad for wartime I 'spose. Sponge cake I made for the babies and jellies with fruit in for all. We had sandwiches, tiny rolls, buns, bread and butter, oh everything. We decorated the dining room with Hugo's aid before he went to bed. Streamers everywhere. He gets about (walking of course) so quickly that it is difficult to keep up with him. He was as cross as two sticks all afternoon and we were terrified he was going to be in a bad mood for the party. However, like his Papa he was charming, very serious but obviously enjoying himself from first to last.

Anyhow at six o'clock Hugo went up to bed and I poured myself a large gin and sat me down in front of the fire to drink to you my love. In fact I had half a bottle (one small one for Nanny). I drank to you my love and to our being together next time. Oh how I did wish you'd been here with me.

Must end now. Oh do you love me darling? I *do* love you so very much and in so many many ways. I think of you all the time and look at my large *Daily Telegraph* map I have on the bedroom wall and wonder just exactly where you are on land or sea.

God bless and keep you my love, my Blackie,
Always and *always* your M.

Margaret to Tam — Halfway Cottage, 8 March 1943

Oh happy Oh sad day,

Three letters from you this morning my darling, written on the boat. How wonderful you are, always when we are apart and you write to me, your letters make me laugh, cry and sometimes think a lot. How strange it must have been for you to stifle all your luxury loving boat habits of a life time, and stifle is the operative word by the sound of the amount of subalterns.

I rang Gwynne to tell her I'd heard and we had a talk about fixing a bike for Loo. She (G) wrote me a very sweet note just after you left saying how she'd hated saying goodbye to you and how miserable she thought I must be etc etc. Nice! For a first wife I thought.

I wonder how many times a day you are conscious of my thoughts? They are with you all the time. I wonder how soon I shall hear from you my love. Oh it will be wonderful when your letters start coming.

Will write again soon my beloved. *Thank you* for the lovely letters my darling. Good night and God bless you for ever,
Your M.

Tam to Margaret — Posted in England, 19 March 1943

My beloved,

This may or may not reach you. I'm relying on a P.T. Sergeant to post it for me on his return. We're nearly there, three or four hours and we dock, so that we can almost say with Walt Whitman[1] 'Oh Captain oh Captain one fearful trip is done.' Except that it hasn't been fearful. The R.A.F. gave us a most courteous welcome about half an hour ago. Two Hurricanes dipped and flew below the level of the deck. Very thrilling. Blue sea and real sun and white villas and that lovely haze on the hills gave me the most painful nostalgia and I became very love sick and depressed. You're so orchidaceous and of the sun that it seemed you must be around somewhere. It was difficult to force oneself back to the unpleasant thought one was entering a theatre of war – it seemed much more as if one was on a rather lonely holiday.

I've just weighed myself in my full equipment – 17 stone 4. We have a march ahead of us this afternoon. I now have to draw an enormous quantity of Bully Beef. The things one does for England, from reciting Shakespeare to housekeeping.

Let the rest of the family know you've had a letter – sorry it's a short one, but I've had an hour to pack, draw rations, water, etc. So it's something of a triumph to have got one off. Morale here is *very* high and there's a laugh a minute. God bless you all my darlings,

Tam

1. Tam is remembering the opening line 'Oh Captain, my captain, our fearful trip is done', from 'Leaves of Grass' by Walt Whitman.

Margaret to Tam — Halfway Cottage, 9 March 1943

Well my angel darling,

Had to write to you tonight for your lovely racing starts tomorrow at Windsor. Hugo has told me that I can go on one condition only, that I take him too. Well, he is a bit young and anyhow I told him we must all go together for his first time and it must be Goodwood on a bright clear day with the tents, the dear stuff, the sea, the little girls in their silk frocks and the lovely clean countryside and the smell of horses who have been trying like mad to win their race for chaps like you and me darling.

I sometimes wonder how cross with me you were that day you asked me to marry you. Very, I think. Anyhow so many really miserable things have happened since one wonders how one could ever have been angry about such a thing as your girl getting pissy on the downs with your best friend and missing the first race, but I was a bit frightened I think. Ye Gods we did have fun coming back in the taxi didn't we? So very mad about each other.

When I'm writing to you I sort of isolate myself in the midst of all these women[1] and it is understood that *no* one speaks to me. On the whole we've got on very well indeed. I just keep saying to myself be tolerant, you've got Tam and Hugo which is 100% more than most; and it works.
God bless, take great care, your M.

1. Margaret's mother Ruby lived with her, and Joyce Singleton the home help was frequently around, as were Tam's mother Silver and Margaret's friends Jasmine Bligh and Eliza Clyde.

Margaret to Tam Halfway Cottage, 10 March 1943

Another Glorious Morning, I feel like a leper who has been cured, a doctor with a new degree, an actress in a success, a mother with a new baby, a bird on the first morning of Spring, a woman who has won the Gold Cup or you when you turn up 'Le Grand'. And all because this morning, Wednesday, a piece of official bumf arrived from G.H.Q. saying 'Dear Sir or Madam etc etc etc Tam is *safe* and *well*!!!' I call that plu bloody perfect and now I can start to worry about your O.B.E. NO MORE. I shall finish this letter later, I am so happy but I must also work.

Later

Perhaps I'm not as happy as I started on page one, you are not here. So what the hell have I got to go on about. But at least I can look forward to your letters arriving now. Perhaps with any luck you'll find some of mine waiting for you on arrival.

Hugo is really asserting himself these days! He was off to the Palmers Arms this evening I'm sure, but fortunately he found the gate shut. Bless his heart, he looks very like you sometimes and I love it.

I'm off to fill the bottles, heat Mummy's milk and feed the boy. I suppose that sounds like heaven to you now darling, but I'll take Bermuda or Capri with you anyday. So my love goodnight and I'll see you soon soon soon. Maybe tonight?
For ever always and always,
Your own M.

Tam to Margaret North Africa, 14 March 1943

My Darling,

We disembarked[1] rather thankfully (it seemed at the time fearfully crowded on the ship but really I suppose it was the last bit of comfort we shall see) and marched, mercifully only a mile or so, to a transit camp. Signs along the road were 'To Transit Camp and Dumps' which is charmingly worded and extremely accurate. It turned out to be the State Municipal – empty bathing pools (the drunks all fell in the deep end coming home in the dark) and the football ground. The troops sleep in the Grandstand. The evening we arrived they were wonderful – cold and strange and not having had very much to eat, sitting in the grandstand with one blanket for the night, they invented an imaginary football match, and for an hour or so there was continual applause and shouting into the darkness remarks and instructions to the Referee and players. Whoever started it must be a great man – humour triumphed over discomfort and homesickness, and they were as happy as kings. Then some Welsh Fusiliers began singing 'Men of Harlech', 'All Through the Night', and 'Land of My Fathers', and I finished the last drop of my whisky and went emotionally to my camp bed quite convinced that Englishmen are magnificent because they're slightly mad.

Our second day here was my birthday – we dined in the town extremely badly. Five courses. Cabbage soup followed not very surprisingly by cabbage as the second course. The third was artichokes and tinned peas, the fourth a passable omlette [*sic*], and the fifth a tangerine. The wine coloured the teeth and scented the lips so that cigarettes tasted as though they'd been in your bag. I made a note of them. The white was Miliana Monnier. Rue Valentin. Tel: 32927. The red Mellea – Extra Vieux. Maison Montserrat, tel: 28733. I shall ring them up from New York sometime and tell them to fuck themselves.

I'm now Intelligence Officer at Squadron headquarters,[2] which should make Johnny laugh himself crimson. Everybody seems incredibly optimistic about the campaign and I'm more certain than ever it's going to be like Ascot on Friday – with considerably more interest being taken in the next meeting, if you know what I mean and I think you do.[3] One of the things that keeps my own morale up is the feeling at last one is on the spot. Everyone here says the French have fought magnificently (and the Guards) and one splendid little Welsh subaltern in the Parachutes with an M.C. and a Medale Militaire, who thought quite obviously they weren't nearly as much to be proud of as playing in *One of Our Aircraft is Missing*, told me there were three people he took his hat off to – 'Bloody terrific man' – and they were the Transport Drivers, the Gunners and the Pioneer Corps. By the way, did I tell you that censoring some of the letters on the ship I came across the following – 'You remember Elsie always said I was like Hugh Williams – well she wouldn't if she could see him face to face like I have – he's quite old with gray hair.'

I've just heard I'm off again ahead of the others, there must be something about my face which suggests advance parties.[4] Farewell Civilisation. Saw Jack Profumo[5] on the way back last week who produced an enormous Gin and said 'Tell Margaret to give my love to everyone, there's nothing to do with it out here.' I think this is enough – can't write after sunset – we've no light. My love to my Hugo and Nannie – and you my beloved forever and ever and always and always,
Tam

1. Tam disembarked at Algiers.
2. Tam was serving with Phantom's 'K' Squadron, which was liaising with American forces under the command of General Patton, who was preparing an attack on Gafsa.
3. Tam is referring cryptically, due to the censor, to the fact that people were less concerned with events in North Africa than with the longed-for invasion of Europe.
4. Phantom's main function was to dispatch patrols to forward positions so that they could report back to headquarters on the movements of those in the front line, and the enemy's responses to these. Thus it was hoped to prevent troops in the rear firing on their own side further forward.
5. John Dennis Profumo OBE, born 1915, served in the First Northamptonshire Yeomanry during the war. Afterwards he became a Conservative Member of Parliament and Cabinet Minister, but resigned after lying to the House of Commons about his affair with Christine Keeler.

Margaret to Tam Halfway Cottage, 20 March 1943

My love my Tam,

As I read your letters and enjoy them I can't help envying the censors the enjoyment they must get – *and before me*. Your description of the blue sea and sunshine made me feel very drab, pale and foggy darling, and I feel we should never be apart in the sun, for you and I are both at our best in a warm climate. You also said in your letter that I am orchidaceous; I wish you could see me now after ten days solid of young Mr Hugo. However, we are good – really good friends now and have been very happy together.

With your letter this morning arrived a large box and inside, wonder of wonders – a grapefruit, 8 oranges and 10 LEMONS. Thank you so much, golly what a joy. I'd forgotten what lemons and grapefruit looked like.

Spoke to Gwynne the other day. We are a strange menage, but it is so much nicer and easier this way, how I hope it lasts. No fusses and no petty quarrels. I hope it has made you happy darling. For so long you seem to have had so many worries and big responsibilities, it is good to feel I can take care of them for you for a while.

The first of April will see me the proud and moderately happy owner of 6 hens. So now perhaps we'll get an egg or two. Just being here is not really very great news value. Oh, I know, David tells me he is now with D.P.R. (Director of Public Relations). Very cushy, mostly living at home doing some writing etc., but as his boss is ill now he just stays at home because he does not know what to do. Hey hoe! The ever so gallant Mr Niven.

Silver says she will be here April 1st. Bless her. We'll have lots of fun and talks together, we have one great thing in common, our love for you darling.

Goodnight, God keep and bless you my Blackie, always and always,
Your own M.

Tam to Margaret North Africa, 21 March 1943

My darling darling Margaret,

I was sent on in advance with this jeep to deliver to E Squadron[1] and I'm waiting here for our own lot. In the two weeks since landing I must have travelled something like 1700 miles. Grand trip up this time but poor weather – rainy and bloody cold in the mountains. I shall see if I can send you through a message. Get Johnny to get hold of the messages you can send back. 'Always and always' I'm afraid is impossible, one has to stick to the sort of 'My love and thoughts forever with you dearest'.

It appears to me I have at last discovered a place it is impossible to spend money – it is unfortunate it should be in a rather muddy waddy in Tunisia, however there is every chance I shall not spend my 2400 frs per month. Yesterday for instance I purchased eight new laid eggs for twenty four cigarettes from something which in the half light of dusk appeared to be a large goat – but when it counted the cigarettes out loud I presumed to be an Arab. I mix French and Italian – not Vermouth – and they seem to understand admirably.

How strange to be sitting here listening to an English sky lark singing – it is Sunday morning and I might so easily be under the plum tree by the pram. Give Hugo a kiss on the back of his neck for me and a lump of chocolate to wipe all over his chin for being able to walk – please God he'll never have to march – I think of him so much.

The other night three Paratroopers passed me in the street and then ran after me. They had done the jump on the airport in Tunis way back in December, and had just come out of hospital. They were some of the boys who had worked in *Secret Mission*[2] last May. We had several bottles of Glyco Thermolyne[3] together. And a Traffic Control chap asked me for my autograph on a mountain road 5000 ft. up in the Tel Atlas Mountains.[4] I'm afraid I really do enjoy being recognised here, it suddenly restores the balance.

I think it's a pity that Bogus Major[5] has moved next door.

Kiss my daughters for me. I shall love you till I die my own beloved and most valuable wife.

Always and always,
Tam

1. E Squadron was another unit of the Phantom Regiment.
2. *Secret Mission* was one of the films Tam made while on release from active duty in 1942.
3. A type of anti-freeze. Tam is presumably referring to the local hooch.
4. The Atlas Mountains shadow the coast of North Africa (see map). Tam's exact location at this time is unclear.
5. David Niven, whom Tam disliked.

Margaret to Tam — Halfway Cottage, 24 March 1943

Darling darling,

Had a long letter from Jacqueline Deniham, your devoted and ugly fan. I wrote to her and told her you were abroad etc, in fact I've dealt with a lot of your fan mail – and she wrote a sweet letter back with the usual invitations to go to see them. She also enclosed two small hearts on a chain for me to wear until your return and a photograph of us on our wedding day – awful – for us to sign. Oh dear, that photograph made me very sad. It was such a desperate time for England and France but so glorious for Hugh and Margaret. Such extremes of emotions. How happy we were that June day and yet the world of the politicians was clanking and crashing almost in our eardrums. The little people of the world like you and me I suppose will always be the same – I wonder – loving and hating and fighting, while the world's events go surging through and over them. I do write rot perhaps darling, but do you know at all what I mean?

[Continued] Monday 29 March, evening

Wonderful news today, at 2 p.m. the B.B.C. interrupted their programme with a special communiqué to say that Mareth[1] has been taken by the Eighth Army and that Rommel is in retreat. Very exciting and Oh God I shall pray for his extermination and with as little loss to ourselves as it is within His power.

Johnny watched over Hugo for fifteen minutes on Sunday and after he'd turned the radio off twice, pulled a vase of daffodils over and pulled all the papers off the desk, Johnny came out to me with a desperate expression on his face and Hugo under one arm and begged me to come back, said he'd rather have three Phantom squadrons to look after.

Have to learn to use a violin for this film[2] and let me tell you my love, it is *bloody difficult*, I have a lesson every other day and practise in odd moments. I just *will* do it right, but it really is tiring, the position one has to get into is not nearly as easy as it looks. Thank goodness I start work soon, finance is getting a bit tricky. But I'm O.K. I promise.

All these bits of news seem supremely unimportant when I think of today's news and what it might mean. Oh my love, remember June 21st, I wonder, I wonder. I feel as if you've been gone for years and it's not yet six weeks. I feel like a clock without any jewels, a flower with no scent, a sky without the blue, or just me without you. It just sometimes makes me feel like a fool for bothering to go on without you about, and then I pull myself together and tell myself that I must get on with it and try to help you by being halfway decent here and making our family happy and comfortable while you are away. I do love you so tremendously darling. Take care of yourself and remember that I'll love you always whatever happens.

Goodnight and God bless you my Blackie,
Forever and always, your own M.

1. After defeat at El Alamein in November 1942 the Germans retreated to Tunisia. Knowing that they couldn't invade France until North Africa was entirely under their control, the Allies pursued them, and General Montgomery took Mareth in the first decisive victory on Tunisian soil on 26 March 1943.
2. *The Lamp Still Burns*, 1943, directed by Maurice Elvey, starring Stewart Granger, Cathleen Nesbitt and Joyce Grenfell.

Tam to Margaret North Africa, 30 March 1943

Early morning – or what in happier times was late at night. Strong and sweet black coffee laced with the last little drop out of my flask. I've just dressed myself under extreme difficulties. Inside a very dark tent to find each garment strewn on the bed required a flick of my lighter. It having rained for eight hours (the rainy season having finished last week), the ground was like any car park at any Saturday race meeting in mid winter, and to balance on a camp bed in outer darkness to avoid the inches of mud was too much for me. A foot – with the sock on it unfortunately – went in. I think it was only yesterday I complained of the dust. On the way through the cactus and the fig trees I fell into a large hole which I'm now beginning to think was a latrine a month back during the enemy occupation of this so charming oasis. The battle seems to be going well – these Allies of ours take it very steady after dark and there's nothing much coming in. Good news from Monty[1] today. Quite chilly at night and my lamb lining is a Godsend but you might tell your furrier I fancy the majority of his customers would prefer him to remove the pins before delivery. I've already extracted three and lost a considerable amount of blood. My lavatory seat is another blessing – crouching made my legs very stiff and my braces damp. In fact, I find on the whole my wardrobe and etceteras were wisely chosen.

I'm still floundering in the work. Nothing could be more difficult than to start operations with the Americans – I know very little of our own army but absolutely fuck nothing about theirs. I wake sometimes, which is foolish considering how little I sleep, and lie sweating with anxiety wondering whether my map is marked correctly or if I've forgotten some vital information. I lose notebooks and have to rely on little bits of paper and an indifferent memory. But it's stupid of me to say floundering for this is only the first week and I'm learning all the time. The trouble is the campaign will finish before I become even moderately efficient. What then? I wonder.

I think a great deal about immediate post-war entertainment. What will the dear dear Public want? A love story with a gay smart background. Not of the war, yet it would be impossible to exclude it – so what – a reunion of lovers or husband and wife – which is tricky, which is sentimental, which is amusing, which is finally completely happy. Happiness. Let us have a play about happiness. No one has had more than a nod from happiness for so long – except you and I Beloved. We must have something that does not

tax the intelligence. And we must have a teensy weensy touch of a better world and better understanding. I know the ingredients so well but I'm as barren as this Goddam desert of ideas. Anyway, whatever it is I shall be dressed superbly – in fact I think I shall be pretty bloody exquisite for quite some time after this war – silks and lotions and elegant pin stripes and long sessions at the barber, and frequent massage, but not until you my loveliness have run amok in every milliner and salon from Knightsbridge to Regent St. How wonderful you'll look my darling – and every morning I shall telephone the florist to acquaint him with the colour for the day and for the evening, and never again will a red carnation be made to last from lunch till the following dawn. A run in the stocking my pretty will not concern you for you will be wrestling with weightier problems, maybe you will have difficulty in deciding between caviar and avocado, maybe you will be wishing to cancel a fitting in order to take me to bed around 3.30 – maybe you will be worried because the dear stuff is no older than your son. The cut of a coat or the setting of a diamond may concern you but never again a ladder in your stocking. And by God I'll have my shoelaces washed every day. So you see my interest in post-war drama is not entirely without a distressing commercialism, for I intend no longer to practice this foolish and half-hearted method of letting money slip through my fingers. That is slipshod and haphazard. I intend, in future, to allow it to pour in a great torrent from as many pockets as my tailor will permit me. Don't be alarmed my darling, this is only the talk of a man with mosquito ointment on his face and hands and anti-louse powder in the seams of his clothing, who drinks his highly medicated morning tea from a tin mug with shaving soap on the rim and uses Gum Boots for bedroom slippers. There is a little noise going on – I must see why. Our allies fire their pistols at aircraft flying at any altitude irrespective of nationality in the most reckless 'Give 'em all you've got boys' manner. You won't believe me but it's true. I like Americans – 'Perhaps you'd like to share my candy?' said a Brigadier this morning. What Englishman of that rank would ever give a subaltern a peppermint lifesaver? My love forever, and much more when there's time,
Tam

1. Tam is referring to Montgomery's victory at Mareth on the south-eastern coast of Tunisia (see map).

Tam to Margaret North Africa, 4 April 1943

My darling,

I am amazed more than appalled by the hours one works and how long one can go without sleep when teetotal. What a wonderful party Hugo must have had. Oh dear, oh dear, I hate missing things like that. Springett has done very well, took 41 Italian prisoners,[1] not exactly Phantom's job but he gets touchy with our Allies. Sent you a message earlier this week asking for corduroys. Sorry but they're essential. Also fly papers and fly swatters. Lux is that possible? Also would it be too much to open your next large tin of soup by making a small hole, refilling with whisky, solder up and dispatch! This merely an idea I had driving along a terrible road the other night – bitterly cold. Hit a camel in the back legs going very fast, didn't stop as I remembered they bit you sometimes. My beloved you shall have a decent letter soon, really too busy at the moment. Yours are a Godsend – but disturbing, oh how disturbing. Pray for the Russians, they've got to beat Germany – if not – Christ – I don't know, I really don't. Take care of yourself. I love you so much my darling, God bless you – stay loving me. Always and always,

Tam

1. Dick Springett was awarded the Silver Star by the Americans for this action.

Margaret to Tam Halfway Cottage, 5 April 1943

My own beloved,

On Friday Silver and the girls arrived, poor old Silver very exhausted but the girls radiant. Loo is slimmer and if possible prettier and Prue bless her much fatter and looking wonderful. They were really sweet to me. I think I've overdone the not touching them or kissing them except at bedtime. I've always been petrified they'd think I was mauling them, but they really were very affectionate, gay and sweet.

Sunday Ye Gods how frightened I was – Gwynne and Silver and the girls and Mummy and Nanny and Hugo all in the house for the night. But the whole thing went off very well without an awkward moment or hitch. We talked, had tea, then the girls did a little scene from Shakespeare they learnt themselves and produced for themselves. It really was *enchanting* and they did it all as if they really understood the words they spoke. Even when Niven and Prim arrived as they were about to begin they only made a slight demur and went on with it. Loo of course was lovely and full of grace, but little Prue suprised me by being very funny and much more full of character. We had a jolly little drink then Gwynne and I gave them a very merry giggly bath and put them to bed.

I can't find the Tel Atlas mountains on my map, but have a *fair* idea of where you are. I'm thinking of you by your tent with the sun shining on you and your drying pyjamas waving in the breeze. Take care of yourself darling and always remember every moment of every day that I'm loving you and planning for our lovely years together.
Always my beloved and always your own wife, M.

Tam to Margaret Tunisia, 8 April 1943

My beloved,

Oh my oh my! What a busy and exciting day. Remember back when you get this and work out what we've been working on.[1] Did very well. It really is very thrilling. But sometimes I wonder if when it's over we'll be glad or shall we think I was a fool to sacrifice so much and so many? Oh God we'll be glad, won't we? I don't know. Not in this Goddam dust hurricane I don't. You and Hugo have a thick coating of desert on your faces – I must wipe you. The mosquito net is blowing about like a mad khaki ghost and the wind in the fig trees is getting louder. Bed now, which will be rather like getting into pyjamas and going to sleep in a Bunker.
God bless you my angel,
Always and always,
Tam

1. Tam's unit was attached to the 8th Army led by General Montgomery, with part of which he marched southwards from the landing site at Algiers to Fériana and Gafsa. His squadron was then seconded to the American 1st Army engaged in heavy fighting around Mejez el Bab (see map).

Tam to Margaret Tunisia, 10 April 1943

I suppose no English soldier ever went abroad since the beginning of our Island history without giving voice to his longings. At Agincourt it was 'I would give all my fame for a pot of ale and safety' and three hundred odd years later in Gafsa it is 'Christ wot I could do to a bleeding pint.' The common soldier doesn't alter much through the centuries and I'm not quite so certain I admire him as much as I thought I did. Shakespeare drew them as appalling line shooters, seeking to impress their friends by growing beards and boasting of dangers they had never faced. Censoring letters is an unpalatable dreary business, but it is very enlightening – there is quite a universal and unanimous note of cheerful gallantry and indifference to discomforts and danger which is rather nauseating. Not one of them has the honesty or – far more important – the human kindness to admit to his dearest that he is disgracefully safe. But there we are, some little woman in some part of England is made proud so what the hell.

The battle – if one can dignify such a stagnant shambles by such a name – in this sector is closed – and there is an atmosphere of clearing away the ashtrays and counting the broken glasses. The dust storm continues, one scrapes it from the bacon fat at breakfast, one sees it at the bottom of the mug of tea, it is in one's tooth powder and shaving brush, the ink, the bed, between the teeth and in the throat, inside boxes that are locked and upon dead flies on the fly paper. Several kilos of it are inside my watch which no longer goes. It's like living in a tee box. Someday someone will take me out and drive a Silver King from the top of my head straight down the Fairway.

Goodnight my love and thank you for being everything you are and doing everything you're doing, and if that little boy tires you tie him up in a tree.

Next morning

Saxin[1] before I forget it. Had a very steady night. I'm just off to what was the battlefield to see what there is in the way of loot. A bit carrion-like, but we need odds and ends. I like to think of you and Gwynne spending a weekend together. It proves what fundamentally nice people we all are, and how we all admire each other and have one common goal – to see our children launched into the pomps and wickedness of the world as safely as we can. God knows what they make of it. Anyway, I think you're wonderful. Strike at Two Gates cottage[2] while the bounce is still in the cheques.
Tam

1. This was a form of sweetener which Tam wanted Margaret to send out to him.
2. The lease was up on Halfway Cottage and Margaret was entering into negotations to rent a smaller house in Dorney village.

Margaret to Tam Halfway Cottage, 16 April 1943

Well my most beloved,

David and Prim had their christening today[1] with banners and stars flying. Vivien and Larry[2], Diana and Carol Reed[3] and the inevitable Trubshaw[4]. Only heard about it from Tommy Clyde who is at home waiting for Eliza's baby to appear. I was *not* invited, in spite of the fact that they were here *plus* their house party the weekend before last. Bloody rude, and after the way he lived off you in Hollywood I think pretty cheap. Not enough alcohol for a Williams I suppose!!!

The country sounds quite lovely and of all the news and talks one has heard from North Africa, suprising that no one has yet mentioned its beauty. But perhaps that does not go with their idea of war.

Golly your description of the football match in the darkness of that place on your first night made me cry. Darling how could such men ever fail? But the saddest bit was that you'd finished your whisky. Would there be any chance of your getting it if I sent a bottle? *Please tell me.*

Another perfect day, deep blue sky, not a cloud in sight and hot sun. Very odd for so early in April, but so so lovely darling I feel you have sent it to me. Your second parcel of fruit arrived last Friday my love – wonderful dates and oranges for Hugo.
More tomorrow. I'll love you always and always,
Your M.

1. David and Primula's first son, David Junior, born 1942.
2. Vivien Leigh and Laurence Olivier.
2. Carol Reed the film producer and his wife.
3. Michael Trubshaw, actor.

Tam to Margaret Tunisia, 16 April 1943

My darling, lovely and most needed wife,

The battle seems to be entering the final stages,[1] very interesting. ALL the years of messing around in England I never imagined anything could be anything else but so bloody dull it was unbearable, but I must say it's intensely interesting now it's real.

It's my afternoon off so I'm taking it easy. When I've finished this I shall lie naked in the sun, and then I shall have a sort of a kind of a bath in an aluminium cooking thing I bought in Algiers and then I shall fill my flask and walk over to Jack P.'s and give him a drink. I'm running the Mess now. A bloody job but I announced before I took it that I had no intention of running it honestly – so I've managed another bottle of whisky for myself and I get more chocolate now and I've a slight pull with airgraphs.

Sharing a tent now with John Hoskyns, the signals officer, a nice boy, has great advantages. Telephone, radio (Tommy Trinder[2] tonight) and our own electric light.

My morale is high – not much longer here I don't think, and if we can mount our invasion of Europe this summer and the Russians have another big crack this winter[3] we should have them in the bag. And then, my darling, then – dear God what joy. I should like to have a very good tea now and take you to bed. My lesser Celandine you'd look so lovely in the sunshine – your long body brown and golden. Instead what? You're feeding the chickens and bathing the baby and I'm on duty this evening. Sometimes it seems we love England more than each other, the things we do for her. God bless you my darling, take care of yourself. I shall love you always and always,
Tam

1. The 8th Army was still advancing northwards towards Tunis.
2. Tommy Trinder (1909–89), comedian.
3. The Russians were still fighting the Germans in Eastern Europe but the Allies could not effect the crucial invasion of France until North Africa was taken and the necessary troops made available.

Margaret to Tam — Halfway Cottage, 23 April 1943

Tamèd my beloved,

You sound fairly comfortable darling, under the circs. I'm worried about that old pain in your back coming again. Can you get Phensic?

In my last long letter I told you that I was about to start work. Started on Wed. Not a bad day and everyone was very sweet to me, had to do my stuff with the violin, very nervous, but they seemed quite pleased. It is a hell of a thing to do really, and when it is all cut up I suppose very little will remain really. Bob Newton[1] is working with Celia[2] and John Mills in *This Happy Breed*. They all sent you their love, specially Celia!! Bob looking very fat and very much on the waggon!!! I think Celia has him under control.

Another lovely box of lemons from you this week, also one for Silver which I'll take up to her on Mon or Tues.

My time when I'm alone is all spent now (my great luxury) in making and dreaming plans for us darling, of all the lovely things we'll do and say to each other in the years to come. I don't think I'd ever really realised what a wonderful bit of luck it was for me the day I finally trapped you. I only want to make you happy now. Oh God how I think and think and think of you and miss you my beloved. But I'm alright, in fact we all are and in some odd way we are able to be fairly happy without stopping to think too much, and I suppose you are the same. Do you *like* being messing officer? Even if you are not honest I should have thought there was very little to be dishonest about.

Another full moon last night darling. I went into the garden and sent lots of messages to you with her. Did you get them I wonder, or did she give them to someone else?
I'll love you always and always,
Your own M.

1. Robert Newton (1905–56).
2. Celia Johnson (1908–82).

Tam to Margaret — Tunisia, 23 April 1943

Yesterday the heavens opened and water fell out. Tents flooded, everything wringing wet and mud everywhere. 'I've never seen rain like it' remarked everyone with more than usual accuracy. Splashing on the roof of the tent it reminds me of Wimbledon. 50/- a ticket no play. 3/6 for tea and the strawberries run out. Had a bottle of beer – I suppose it was filthy but it tasted magnificent. The water lately has been highly flavoured. This is a stupid sort of letter but how to make it otherwise? Privacy is the essential thing in correspondence. I've no intention of having my affection first photographed and then reduced in size. What happens then I don't recollect. Maybe it will be flung on the Silver Screen at the Slough Granada in mistake for 'Is there a Doctor in the House?' So give my kind regards to Hugo, yours very sincerely,
Tam

Tam to Margaret — Tunisia, 24 April 1943

It's strange to be leading a life entirely without either comfort or pleasure. I'm not grumbling for as I say one's enormously lucky, but having taken a great deal of trouble all one's life to seek pleasure, to find now delights are down to a borrowed Benzadrine taken in chlorinated water is strange. No doubt excellent for one. And there are your letters and the weather and the views, and the lights in the evening and the wild flowers, and now there is bread and no longer those Army Biscuits that have been made from the road-blocks we didn't need in 1940. And during the busy moments the excitement is terrific – nothing was ever quite so terrific. And there are the times of looking forward and the times of looking back. Ta ta for now, something's come in.

That was yesterday, now it's Easter morning. Just been to early service in the Conference tent with the noise of our Bombers overhead as a running commentary on the stupidity of man. We could hear shelling the other night. I don't know if I'm a fool or over conscious of the dramatic values – an actor's failing I've always guarded against – but I lie in bed and wonder morbidly what kind of men are being killed – for what reason and for how long – and if they've sons and daughters.

Naturally as we've just got our Tropical kit it's been cold for the last few days, and wet.

Jack Profumo is a few yards away in a most luxurious office truck with pictures of lovelies all over the walls.

Darling I think such an awful lot about all the things you're doing to keep the family united. Those girls will adore you by the time they're twenty. Would I have been proud of them acting *The Dream* in the garden?

Afraid my letters are very disjointed, so many interruptions.

Always and always,

Tam

Margaret to Tam — Halfway Cottage, 27 April 1943

Tamèd my Tam,

Each time I sit down to write to you my poor little brain is so seething with things I want to say to you and questions I want answered that I sometimes wonder if my letters make any sense at all. Yours of course are wonderful my darling and I almost live on them. They are read and re-read until I almost know them by heart. I've sent you a parcel sweetheart of razor blades, a nail file, a pillow slip and 2 prs of garters, which I do hope are the sort you want, they look very odd but the man assured me that they were the thing and that they are very hard to get now – elastic I suppose! Your corduroys are on their way, I nearly sent you a pair of natty green ones but I thought you'd be *safer* in sand colour.

While I think of it – I read in the paper today that the word Tunisgrad is being scrawled on walls and hoardings in Germany during the night.[1] The descriptions of the fighting going on out there are very frightening now, they sound so desperate and fierce, bayonet charges and hand to hand fighting. Ye Gods darling, how long can it last? Men can't hate hard enough for that sort of thing to last long. Whatever you do, just remember us and know that we (Hugo and I) love you and think of you all the time darling.

Johnny told me that Dick Springett had heard that the Huns had some whisky and as supplies were low with him he went over to get some and caught 40 prisoners. Is it true? Wonderful if it is. Also I hear there are good reports of you my love, but *please* no bravery and if you do hear they have some wine 'over there' just remember that it might be corked!

Tell Jack P. that I've practically given all his love away, and give him my best. Just a few days before I got your letter saying you'd seen him I met his brother at the Clydes. He told me that Jack had been run over by a tank but was O.K. again. From all I can gather the bogus Major next door has made himself quite a wide range of enemies from opening his big mouth too wide. You know the way he chats on about himself. The latest is he has been offered a job to take over a certain squadron out there, but he is still gardening madly in Dorney. Miaow!!

Perhaps there may be a letter from you in the morning, hope you are getting all mine beloved. I love you more than anything or anyone in the whole wide world. You are part of me and my very own always and always. Sometimes it is bad, I want you so much for so many reasons. Good night, God bless and keep you for me,
Your own M.

1. Linking the Allied capture of Stalingrad with their successes in Tunisia in a bid to demoralize the Germans.

Tam to Margaret Tunisia, 28 April 1943

Was on duty last night and have just had a magnificent bath. Sitting in a canvas bag with my legs outside in a tin basin – the water was moderately clean and free from tiny little fish and I was profligate with Algerian Eau de Cologne. Clean clothes now and I feel wonderful. There is something rather charming about picking a wild flower as you sit in your bath and having an uninterrupted view for twenty miles right down a valley which looks like a painter's palette – great patches of crimson poppies – blues and yellows and lavenders – shadows and sunlights. I sat there and felt very in love and quite amazingly happy.

Another interruption, a sort of transient army barber appeared at the entrance of my tent – I discovered just as he was finishing my hair that he was a stone mason in Bristol. To think the word tent once suggested to me great barrels of ice with the gold tin foil on the corks just keeping their pretty heads above water, or the setting Shakespeare chose for Brutus and Cassius to play the greatest quarrel scene ever written, or an overpowering and exhausting day in Regent's Park for the Garden Party. 'Who's that?' 'Oh we don't want him' 'Where's Ivor?' And now it's my world.

Don't like this Russian-Polish rumpus[1] – can hear nothing but the castrated news the B.B.C. delivers – but am filled with alarm – it may cause THE most fearful trouble. Pay no regard to the B.B.C. news of this theatre, it's mostly Phantom stuff and they have trouble in reading Hugh Fraser's[2] writing. Pamphlets in German saying 'Lay down your arms – it is useless' have been dropped in error outside the C–in–C's tent – which lends colour to the dull daily routine.

Mother tells me in her letter of the most Magic April since the war began – I'm afraid you'll have trouble with me later – I begin to feel like Browning in April and long for the bloom and blossom of England. God bless my darling and my Hugo – a kiss on the back of his neck and an extra few minutes in the bath for him. But for you my beloved my entire heart. Always and always.
Tam

P.S. The forty ninth moon is coming up now. How many more I wonder?

1. On 26 April the Germans uncovered a mass grave of 4,000 Polish officers near Katyn and claimed they were murdered by the Russians. This caused serious friction between the Soviet Union and the Polish government.
2. Later Sir Hugh Fraser (1918–84). After the war he became a Member of Parliament, and was Secretary of State for Air from 1962–4. He was knighted in 1980.

Margaret to Tam — Halfway Cottage, 5 May 1943

My Precious Beloved,

Glorious glorious week, up to today I've opened seven letters from you so I've been living in a wonderful daze of happiness. How I love your letters, they are so full of you, and I know it may sound silly, but I *do* think you are wonderful. Your letters are full of your old spark of humour and wit in spite of all the dirt and sand and noise and discomfort that I know you abominate so much. What a God-send it must be for you to be able to see the funny side – or do you? Is it just to make me feel happier about you? Whichever it is I *worship* you my darling and I'm really with you all the time. Don't ever suggest that I'm putting up with any hardships my love. Just ask yourself which you'd rather do – stay here and work and keep our little gaggle fed and warm or be in that bloody sand and filth. *I'm* the one who's going to give you a lovely life after it is all over darling, and don't ever imagine I'm not certain that this is the way it must be. Just keep this letter and if I'm ever bloody minded in years to come tweak it out and show it to me. What ever happens you are *first* forever.

You said you'd like to know if I've been worried or creaky. Well I *have* been creaky but not worried, just a little – shall I say puzzled. However I'm over the worst and I've now seen a spot of the light at the other end of the tunnel. Sold my earrings for £200, not bad, eh?

I've had all of your wonderful letters from the boat, they made quite good time, I heard much sooner than I expected. Will send you fly exterminator and lux and soap this week darling, and hope you have the corduroys and other odds and ends by now.

All my love is always with you my beloved, for ever and ever and please take care of yourself,

Your own M.

Margaret to Tam — Halfway Cottage, 6 May 1943

Well my best beloved,

How to ever tell you how much your letters mean to me, they are wonderful darling and full of you. They make me feel so close to you, almost talking to you. Golly how I'd love to be able to sit and have a huge drink and long talk to you right now. I've been pretty creaky the last few weeks, but now work has started and the money is coming in and I've had £20 from your bank and I've sold my diamond earrings for £200, not bad eh? So now we are alright for a while.

Worked hard all this week. Think they are quite pleased with me so far and I thought I looked quite nice in the rushes. Hair not very good though, must do something about it. So far I've done five days, so should get about twelve out of it with luck.

I've had seven letters of various sorts and kinds from you this week darling. Golly, apart from the dust, bad food and lack of sleep you must be having a pretty interesting time my pet. It is so hard to sit here at our fireside in our little house and realise as we listen to the news that you are actually there in the midst of what one of those B.B.C. poops are telling us about in their flat dull voices. It makes me boil. Oh darlingest I shall make up to you one day with an hour of fun and pleasure for every minute of misery and cold and discomfort you've had in this war. I'll show you just how much I love you one day. You shall have masses of wonderful suits, lovely shirts with your initials on them and exquisite silk pyjamas and dressing gowns and ties – always spotless!! And rows of perfect and polished shoes which you will never walk in ever – only conga occasionally.

Now to answer your questions my love. The first and most important 'Will we be glad?' Darling you *know* we will. We'll have each other for ever and always be able to look each other clearly in the eye and know the right thing was done. I know this for certain when I look around me at the shifty uncomfortable creatures I meet each day, pretending they think they are lucky to be out or ill or whatever they are. But deep down inside they are MISERABLE – they are not in and therefore they will have no share in peace.

I've got your lux, your pipe cleaners and fly papers, but the saxin and fly swatter are proving difficult. But I'll get them. I'll get them. In the meantime I'll send off the others my love. I'm also sending you a bottle of your medicine[1] – see that you take it every evening round 6!!!

Have had letters from 5 out of my 8 welfare chaps'[2] families. Here they are. Tpr Wolfe's sister, who says soap and writing paper seem to be the things he wants. Cpl C. Reeves' sister who's also got a husband in the forces. Gnr S. Walters' wife who says he was right through the last war. She wants to get a small grant to help her pay for a pair of glasses. I think I shall write and ask her how much she wants and if it's not too much I'll fix it for her, poor old girl. Sweet letter from Rfn A.A. Metcalf's father, who tells me that 40 years ago he and his wife courted in this part of the country. They say that their son was at Dunkirk poor boy. And Pte Seel's wife who has only had 2 letters which took six weeks to get to her.

Hugo is cock of the walk in Dorney. He'll have no nonsense from anyone. He's always always busy, never still for a moment and as sturdy and rosy and fit as a fiddle (not the fucker I played on!!)

Goodnight my best beloved, or good morning or good day. They

are all alike away from you. I am loving you every moment of every day.
Always, Your M.

1. Presumably a bottle of whisky!
2. As an officer's wife Margaret was required to keep a friendly eye on the wives of men serving in Tam's patrol, passing on news and giving help where possible.

Tam to Margaret Tunisia, 9 May 1943

It's been good being here – God wot I miss you more every day, that there are a hundred discomforts a day, that there is continual worry and strain and we work like beavers. Everything is checked and checked. (The other night I was tired and bleary eyed and let a message go in locating a Battalion of Americans in the middle of a lake!) I'm glad and I always shall be to have been here. It's occurred to me that you may be wondering, now that this campaign is nearly over, if we're coming home. No. There are plans – I don't know what – but they concern Phantom. We've done very well and our stock is high. So many things happening here I should like to tell you – I will in time. My God the R.A.F. have given them stick. There never seems a moment in the day without the drone of bombers.

Nearly three weeks without a letter from you. It's a balls up with the Army Post Office but the more you send the more will arrive. My love to you all beloved. For always and always, until I can, take care of yourself,
Tam

Margaret to Tam Halfway Cottage, 10 May 1943

My Tamèd,

Just had to write to you today, what brave and glorious news, Tunis and Bizerte.[1] Heard the news early this morning as I was off to the studio. Oh golly I just stood stock still and wanted to cry, and thought of you and wondered just what it meant to us, and for a moment I was bursting with joy because I thought it might mean your coming home soon. But as I drove to the studio through the early morning sunshine I gradually realised that it was pretty hopeless for a while yet. However I've decided that tonight as I sit here writing to you, if you are the man I hope you are, you are getting STINKING in Tunis; but I'm not sure I want you to be with one of those flighty, flirtatious flower-throwing French femmes. Tamèd God of Africa I adore you. Oh dear my beloved do always remember this and take care of yourself, great care.

Was called this morning for 7.45, got there, was washed, shampooed, made up and dressed by about 9.45, went to my room, No 5 (yours I believe), lay down and fell asleep, the phone rang and someone said you can go home darling – the electricians are still on overtime strike. So I took off my finery and came home. Oh dear the things one gets paid for. And now they are paying me £5 a day for my old mink which I'll be wearing in a scene, so I'm trying to think of ways of getting it as many days work as is humanly – or should I say minkably – possible. The next thing is it will be wanting to act!

Silver found her first class digs quite impossible – so the poor old darling has had to move again but she says she *thinks* they have struck lucky this time. The house is called The Haven. Ye Gods the places we've all lived in since the war, particularly you my darling. Gypsy Tam you sound like now my love.

There is nothing much to look forward to tomorrow, no one coming for the week end and I can't hope for a letter until Monday. I love you till I die and long after that,
Always, M.

1. On 8 May 1943 the Allies captured Tunis, then Bizerte (see map).

Margaret to Tam — Halfway Cottage, 14 May 1943

O darling darling,

Had two letters from you this morning and in the one dated May 3rd you said you'd had none from me for two weeks. Golly I'm upset, I've written often and regularly sweetheart, and can't bear to think of you not getting my letters.

Your bath out of doors sounds quite extraordinary and not unlovely with such a view darling, but very hard to imagine. I've always rather wanted to have a bathroom entirely walled by glass, the sort of stuff they have in Paris where you can see out but no one can see in.

By the way, I've already seen to it in several ways that it is known you are abroad, but I shall go further in the matter now darling, now that you've mentioned it.

Niven is looking for a house in Denham, he is going to make some film about the army with Carol Reed directing. Larry is hard at it, testing for *Henry the Fifth* and shaving his hair off and having hair pieces made. Rex,[1] Lilli,[2] John Mills and Rolie Culver[3] are making a film called *English Without Tears* directed I hear by ye dainty French[4]. Larry tells me that Viv and a party of six are going out to Gibraltar and on to Tunisia – golly *I wish I were with them*. They'll be away three months, I gather, so you'll probably see her darling. They all sent great love, and I'm sending you all I possess for always, your M.

1. Rex Harrison.
2. Austrian actress Lilli Palmer (1914–86), Rex Harrison's wife.
3. Roland Culver (1900–84).
4. Harold French (*b*. 1897), actor and director.

Tam to Margaret — Carthage, 18 May 1943

So much to tell you my darling, We're at Carthage – seven or eight miles from Tunis – looking across the bay to the well known Cap Bon peninsula, and everybody is trying to remember the Punic wars, and how Hannibal had a crack at Rome, which all seems very up to the minute but in fact was well over 2000 years ago. He employed elephants as his secret weapon and went up through Spain. Shall we I wonder? I'm in favour of Turkey which I have a strong suspicion is only waiting until the plaudits of victory have died a little – then a pretext and a fairly sensational entrance into the struggle from the prompt corner.[1] Is it appalling or thrilling to know that Alexander[2] is gazing across the same dazzling sea, making his plans for the defeat of Italy from exactly the same spot as Hannibal did in 250 B.C.? It's easy to find both the romance and wretchedness – but for Alexander on top of this hill with the Union Jack flying from his white villa it must be very sweet indeed. The last man to leave Dunkirk following his beaten army – kicked into the English Channel, utterly routed as no English army had ever been routed before, without one single armoured division in England – and now we see the prisoners rolling down every road – one hundred and fifty thousand of them – nearly three times as many as he left in France. If one had the heart and soul of a soldier that must be sweet. It will rank as the most magnificent 'suivi' the world has ever known.

I spend a lot of time marketing for the Mess. Green almonds yesterday which gave my heart an ugly jerk – isn't it extraordinary how the sight of something associated with you appears and there's your face – those eyes and that mouth – both a size larger than the

rest of it. Your hair shining and soft, your elegant nose and the bones and the line of your jaw – and the lovely length of your neck. Is a man less lucky to have such beauty parted from him, than one who has none and can eat green almonds without wanting to cry out loud?
God bless, all my love to you always and always,
Tam

1. Tam seems to favour a pre-emptive strike against Turkey. Actually, after success in Tunisia, the 8th Army invaded Sicily.
2. General Harold Alexander (1891–69), became supreme Allied Commander in the Mediterranean after victory in Tunisia.

Margaret to Tam Denham Studios, 19 May 1943

Well my own beloved,

Here I am, lying in the sun by the river at Denham, one of the usual hold ups on these so-called 'Big' pictures. Oh well another day and the more the merrier I say. I've already had fourteen days, not bad. The sun is really lovely and warm and makes me miss you more than ever.

A lovely air letter from you, but Oh dear, three weeks and no letter from me. Darling I'm really miserable, I shall just have to write even more often and risk repeating myself.

I do so wonder what they'll do with you now that that particular compaign is over. I *am* so anxious to know darling. And incidentally I'm hearing on all sides what a great personal success you've been. Congratulations darling. Oh yes and do get lots of sleep whenever you can, it does build up your resistance. Particularly you, who need so much sleep.

Hugo loved the airgraph drawing you sent him of yourself in the bath. So did I! It really looked quite like you. Who did it? I hear Larry fell out of a tree while trying to catch a cat (no names mentioned!!) the other day – he is now in bed which is holding up *Henry V* a bit. I wonder how many there will be before it is finished?

Goodnight my most beloved. I do so hope my letters have started coming in again now. I've written lots and lots, but from now on I'll put something in the post every day to make sure.
I'll love you for ever my Blackie, always and always your own M.

Tam to Margaret North Africa, 19 May 1943

There's been a slight let-up in censorship and we're now allowed to mention place names so I can tell you whereabouts we've been operating. After the first trip with Tony which was through Constantine to Le Kef, the whole squadron came forward to Fariana [*sic*] – pretty name – where we started working with the Americans. That I think was around March 25th. The fighting moved north, so did we – to near Souk el Abra [see map] working from then onwards with the American 1st army and the French in the north which strained us to bursting point. The patrols weren't so badly off but Squadron H.Q. was flat out. The coders were working the most ghastly hours and considering the difficulties did splendidly. Error crept in once or twice, such as the unfortunate time I allowed the Royal West Kents to advance through a lake. But only a weary voice telephoning said, 'That Phantom? I say you really must keep these people out of the water. We had the Surreys in there yesterday.' On the whole we did very well, and by golly how we worked. From Souk el Abra on to Medjez El Bub for the final coup de grace. That was very exciting. It's far easier too, for good news in battle travels fast and arrives making sense – it's when everything's rather obscure and there's every indication of a bog that the coding goes haywire and there's an electrical storm and the wireless doesn't work. That's when the anxiety begins. Wondering whether to pass a message in when it looks a bit odd – if it's true it's a scoop, if it's phoney there's terrible trouble. Three times the other day we reported Von Arnim's[1] capture, but they wouldn't believe us. And it was wonderful to mark up on the map the 6th and 7th Armed Divisions roaring up the Medjuda valley split arse for Tunis. All the time the R.A.F. were simply plastering the whole front – there was never a moment of the day when there was silence in the sky – I believe that was one of the reasons there was such a very rapid crumble.

Loot of course has been prolific – sitting cosily back at Army H.Q. of course I missed the market, but Springett got God knows what and a brand new Hotchkiss car – the Arabs are having the most terrific harvest, and have enough weapons to mount a large scale revolt. For generations they'll be wearing uniforms, gas masks, army blankets of five or six different countries. They sit on their haunches for hours and hours watching you and you know if you leave your tent unguarded for a minute they'll have the bloody lot. But the children are lovely – a whole gang of them had a sort of jam session where I swam this morning – a rather quick rhythm and obviously dirty for they shrieked with delight at certain verses and looked at me rather coyly.

I'm told the German prisoners are divided into two types – the ones who say 'This is nothing, you've seen less than 3 percent of our army here. We shall win in Russia this year. We shall be free again soon so watch out and treat us well.' Those are the truculent confident fellows. The others are sulky and sullen, they keep saying they'll win, but seem shaken – they're a bit older too. Anyway, there's a hundred and fifty thousand of them in the cages and a very satisfying sight they make.

I went to Tunis, on the 11th I think it was, we'd been in there three days anyway. Somebody boobed rather for there were no restrictions – I suppose the High-Ups thought the troops deserved some fun and so they do, but it was really a shambles. Cup Final night was a garden fête compared to it. English soldiers rolling, reeling, singing, asleep on the pavements and in the gutters at eleven in the morning and the Yanks simply being sick everywhere – a beastly sight with nobody to cope. The Guards are policing it now and it's reasonable. But the first few days were chaotic. I'd stopped at a farm on the way and bought some wine – villainous powerful stuff – which was lucky for the hotels for officers of course had run out so after a quick look round we drove out to Carthage and ate and drank and swam. The first swim in warmth and real sunshine for four years. We lay on the Roman sea wall and basked and listened to the shelling across the bay on the Cap Bon peninsula and the world seemed raving mad.

It's very upsetting to be sitting here in a tent and wondering where and when we shall be striking at the Northern coast of the Mediterranean and to realise that 2000 years ago some other poor miserable soldiers with swords and shields and elephants were sitting on the very exact spot wondering the very exact thing. Their swords and shields and elephants have become tanks and planes and automatic guns but apart from that you couldn't tell the date to within two centuries. If that's what we've learnt, if that's progress and the development of Christianity and civilisation then I think I'd sooner go native on some coral island and count the world well lost. How can one little mingy actor raise a voice of protest? Besides I'm too old and too lazy. But someone must. The real trouble is that so many men like war, like fighting – not the troops but the officers. They love it. They're bloody frightened half the time, they behave superbly, they lead magnificently and they get the only real kick out of life they've ever experienced. Making love, having children, creating anything, travelling, other people, books and the

Arts never touch them – they by-pass the lot. I'm sure of it. I've talked to them. These Cavalry regulars are the worst. They're simply splendid in battle and they discuss the whole thing afterwards at infinite length as though it were a Point to Point and one presumes somewhere inside them there's a minute heart which grieves for friends of a dozen years who've been killed. I pointed out a rainbow to a Major in the 11th Huzzars last night – it was a wonderful rainbow, a complete arc with the ends in the sea, and another somewhat fainter one behind it. He looked at it, turned back to the map and said 'Unreliable climate.' That sort of thing makes me want to dress in pale green and jump into bed with a dozen pansies. Thank God Phantom is different. In fact someday I think we'll carry the Phantom is different too far. It is so very much a private army and the mess is now like The Sporting Club. No one wears anything resembling a uniform – colours and scarves are de rigeur [*sic*]. I'm sent all over the place in search of eggs and asparagus and artichokes, for they insist, quite rightly, on feeding as well as possible. 'I hear they've lobsters at Tabarka' – 'How far's Tabarka?' – 'About a hundred miles' – 'That's alright, take a jeep.' 'Let's have some fresh meat, somebody get a bullock' – We did and a lot of people got diarrhoea. I had an excellent haul of real Danish butter and ham and tomato sauce the Bosche had left and am off tomorrow to the Yanks for coffee. 'Tam we must have coffee after dinner, can't you get some?' I enjoy it a lot. And there's poker every night. And for the first and last and only time in my life I suppose, I find myself incomparably the best player. Profit is easy but payment very deferred. The sea is turning from blue to green (Unreliable ocean) and the sun is sinking and there's a lovely evening light. Hugh Fraser has a theory North Africa is where the earth broke off from the moon. Write to me a lot – I miss you so much and I'm getting utterly weary of only talking to men and being in this bloody army. Don't worry about me I've been shockingly safe all this time, disgracefully so, really. The only danger was the Yanks firing at planes (generally ours) with Tommy guns. Not very accurate.

Once more, all my love,
Tam

1. General Oberst Hans-Jürgen von Arnim was Commanding Officer of the 5th Panzer Army in North Africa.

Tam to Margaret North Africa, 23 May 1943

Things are going to get tricky shortly. Being a Private Army Phantom is always fighting for a job. We're like a lot of actors who've just completed a successful season and are now wondering anxiously about the autumn. It's a matter of complete embuggerance to me, but the keen boys are bothered. God what a country for insects! They get a new set out every day and the flies round my Gammages Commode are real Bomber type. How I long to pull a chain once more. We're still working with four patrols reporting traffic movements and I'm on duty today. They must be getting bored for I've at great trouble just decoded the following:

There was an old actor called Tam,
Who exclaimed when a babe in his pram,
'Lejeune won't chastise me,
Nor Agate despise me,
As long as I keep clear of ham!'

Your letters are the one and only comfort, except for the sea and the beauty of the place. But I'm missing you more and more. I wish we were busy again in a way. Don't be annoyed the Nivens aren't pleasant neighbours, to be ignored by boring people is a mercy from God himself. It's a splendid marriage, a dumb blond and a chatty liar.

More soon beloved, to write to you is the nearest I can get to you, and so when I write I'm happiest.

Always,

Tam

Margaret to Tam Halfway Cottage, 24 May 1943

Well my beloved,

If the paper in these damn air letters gets much worse it won't matter which side you read them on.

Jas arrived back from her family crisis on Sunday and I've persuaded her to stay another week with us. For besides being great fun having her and Sarah[1] here, her maid Jane is a treasure and is doing the cooking which is grand. I wonder have you had any parcels from me yet darling? I've sent you all sorts of odds and ends including a season racing book, and this week I shall send you some more things.

It's Wings for Victory week[2] in the village so no end of garden parties, fêtes, dances and concerts are being held. I've promised to appear in one of the concerts and I've also produced some of the locals in a really outrageously un-funny sketch, which they chose for themselves and insisted on doing. Hey ho the merry – Oh! I hate it all so much when you are not around. Oh I do wonder how you are, how you look, if you still love me and what H.M. will do with you now that that campaign is over. Or is it?

Maurice Elvey and Betty Baron who wrote the epic I've just finished sent me a lovely 'still' of myself with the violin and they wrote on it 'Thank you for a lovely performance', but things like that make me wonder?? I'll probably stink!!

Take care of yourself, I'll love you for always,

Your M.

1. Sarah Johnson, Jasmine's daughter, born in April 1942, an almost exact contemporary of Hugo's.
2. Wings for Victory Week was an annual fund-raising event, presumably in aid of the RAF.

Margaret to Tam Halfway Cottage, 30 May 1943

Well my beloved,

So you are in Carthage. It was wonderful to have your last letter and know exactly where you are for the first time, although I've often had a pretty keen idea. There was a picture in the *Express* today of the Victory Service in the amphitheatre in Carthage. I thought that you would probably have been there and anxiously scanned the blurred faces for yours, but I'm afraid the padre was about the only recognisable one. I shall keep it though and if you were there you'll be able to tell me where you were sitting. My own beloved how I miss you and Oh Golly on these lovely sunny days and long evenings how I long for you to be here, to make plans and bicycle to Monkey Island and Hindhead together, or would we go in our Packard? Yes I think so!

I did my two small sketches last night and I think they went off quite well. *Golly I was nervous*. Had a couple of sweet letters after thanking me for my contributions to things for Victory Week and saying how much they enjoyed themselves etc, but oh dear, I'm glad it's over.

Jas is sitting behind me with a 'Well, come and talk it is my last night' expression on her face. So my most beloved until tomorrow night I'll say goodnight and God Bless and take care

of yourself and remember I love and miss you more than all the world,
Always and always,
Your M.

Margaret to Tam Halfway Cottage, 1 June 1943

My own beloved Tamèd,

I've just written you an air letter but as usual I feel rather frustrated with so little space to say so much in. I wonder how many of my letters you've had at this point. I've had 24 of various sorts and kinds from you and they are almost worn with reading. I do love them so, you really do write wonderful letters darling.

How's your back darling? Better I hope now that you are back in the sea again. Oh how often I think of you swooping about in the warm salt water feeling the sting in your eyes and then the lovely warmth of the sun on your body as you come out onto a rock or sand. It must make up for a lot. 'Spose you are very brown too, eh? You in Carthage, oh golly, wonder where on earth you'll go next – not England I suppose? No! Even if we haven't the sea and the hot sun there are a lot of lovely things in England in the summer, but right now thinking of you without me in the sun of the Mediterranean I can't remember what they are. I only know that I love and miss you more than anyone else in the world. I'll finish this tomorrow.

2 June

Still no news of Cash and Ian.[1] I've only seen them once since she arrived – she is a tricky little bitch isn't she? However I did give them a lovely dinner and was as nice as I knew how, so that is that. But I'm surprised at old Hunter being so graceless. It is my view that as long as you are young, charming and very pretty you can get away with the pose of not liking other women and being rude to them. *But* when you are no longer pretty and your attraction is only in the eyes of those who love you, then for everyone's good the time has come to be nice to other women. What do you think? I must remember this myself in case I'm caught in years to come!!!!

Bloody windy and raining and cold again. April stuff. Must fly now darling to catch the afternoon post. Will write again tomorrow. All my love and Hugo's forever and ever darling, always your own,
M.

1. Ian Hunter (1900–75), actor, and his wife Cash, great friends of Tam and Margaret.

Tam to Margaret North Africa, 3 June 1943

Churchill arrived to address 1st Army a couple of days ago. Very stirring for the setting was so wonderful – the Roman amphitheatre at Carthage – we had front row seats. He looked quite peculiar, like a Disney or a Beatrix Potter creature, and spoke without his teeth. Cigar, V Sign, and all the tricks. His timing was perfect, and when he considered a point needed applause his dumpy little body remained quite motionless, but rather majestic, until it came. Glad I was there. I thought of the night outside Buckingham Palace with Chamberlain smiling peace with honour, and we kidded ourselves there was a chance. Two little suckers so in love and so longing for a tranquil sunny life. It's very sad to think on.

I don't know why but feel restless and rather depressed. Can't find out the form. If we're on the next party – how big it's going to be – where, when. The thought of messing about here indefinitely – training and attempting to keep the men from going nuts rather terrifies me. Fortunately I have my marketing which is endless fun. I was up at 5.30 and was literally the only white person in the place. Did I tell you an old man cried last week when I bought his chicken?

Getting really fearfully hot. The Squadron Leaders are competing with each other about training programmes and there's an increasing stench of bullshit around the camp. An Officers' course and endless lectures. Deadly, quite appallingly deadly. I miss you more and more my darling – time is so precious and it's flying away. Like being in a tube which keeps passing stations you want to get out at. I want to get out at this summer of 1943 and be with you, and I'm getting bored with the people in my carriage, not really but sometimes.

Saw Jack today, first time since the battle – he's giving a dance! How God knows for I haven't heard even a piano since I arrived in Tunisia.

I shall love you for ever for always and always.
God Bless,
Tam

Tam to Margaret North Africa, 9 June 1943

It seems quite a time since I wrote – not long really but time is moving slowly at the moment. Indescribably boring lectures about subjects that could never be of the slightest service to us – merely to give the appearance of work. Oh God that appearance of activity that the military mind insists upon. If there's no work then for Christ's sake have a picnic. I was so peaceful in my mind as long as the campaign lasted – now with no immediate job in the offing – or remote as far as I know – I feel this most fearful waste of time and long to get home. Harrassed again by the old divided loyalties which have been the only part of the war I can honestly say has been bloody for me. Maybe this cinema racket gives one a wrong impression of one's worth. I now feel I'd be better employed at Denham – which is silly for one must do one or the other and not attempt both as I have done.

Half a hundred moons my love, just coming up. And this should reach you for the shortest night[1] to bring you one more year full of gratitude and love and the invitation to continue – shall we go round again my love – and shall we see and touch and hear each other some time during this new year. Dear God I pray so – or shall I return a gray-haired mad man muttering map references into an ill-kempt beard. This is a grumbling letter – a thing I vowed I'd never write to you. But I've changed my wayward little mind. You must be kept in touch with what goes on. Physical fatigue discomfort and dirt I've not exaggerated upon, for they're nothing – but the black depression when it comes must be told. It's lack of anything to put one's mind on, that's all. I can kill flies now by flicking them – as opposed to banging oneself all over. I think they're slower here than the ones at home for it cannot be that I am quicker. How sad about Leslie Howard[2] – a great loss, a really great loss. How's my Hugo – my love to him. But all of it really and all my hopes and plans for you,
Tam

1. 21 June, their wedding anniversary.
2. The actor Leslie Howard (1893–1943) was shot down on a mission between London and Lisbon.

Margaret to Tam — Halfway Cottage, 11 June 1943

My Tam my darling,

Golly what a wonderful long lovely letter from you. And apart from being terribly interesting I think it is one of the best letters I've ever read. Shall keep it over the weekend and send it to Silver on Monday, she'll love it, but I must tell you again how wonderful, amusing and interesting a letter it is darling, thank you, for I know how terribly busy you are and how much time it takes to write a long letter like that. How I'd love to see you pretending to be the Phantom Mess wife.

Popped in to chat to Eliza Clyde for a moment, very depressed because Tommy has just gone back after his leave. Everyone has a feeling now, and it is probably groundless, that each leave will be their last. Still I suppose something will burst somewhere soon. Wonderful news today about Pantellaria.[1] Johnny says you may have moved – wonder where to? I do so worry about you darling. Keep in touch as much as possible won't you, on account of you are very precious to Hugo and me. We've got lots of lovely memories to live on until we are together to make more. I'll be there on the spot waiting for you just as I've always been,
Always and always,
Your M.

1. On 9 June the Allies began an assault on the Italian island of Pantellaria.

Tam to Margaret North Africa, 11 June 1943

A letter from you yesterday – some of your letters end up because you say someone wants you to talk to them.[1] If this were not going to be photographed I could express myself adequately. To the duck pond with them. Down into the green slime with the mud and the reeds in their eyeball sockets – spongy and stinking from stagnant water – there they should remain as a warning.

How's my Hugo? Shirts and trousers! Poor little Curtis.[2] Another year or so and our Haberdasher accounts will be getting muddled and I shall find myself involved in white waistcoats I've never seen. Tell him he has got to pay cash.[3] Go and tell him now! The thought terrifies me. Write to me a great deal please my pretty. Boredom is setting in, and so discontent and so homesickness and so wretchedness and so all my love to you. Miss you so much. God bless.
Tam

1. Refers to Margaret's letter of 30 May: 'Jas is sitting behind me with a "Well, come and talk it is my last night" expression on her face.'
2. Tam's shirtmaker.
3. Tam doesn't want Hugo's clothes credited to his account.

Tam to Margaret North Africa, 16 June 1943

Two letters from you yesterday. A plague of caterpillars is this month's insect world selection. Six in my shirt this morning – long furry ones with soft centres. Fear my last letter was a misery –

hangover. Better now and am feeling splendid again. Entertained some of the locals last night. Butcher, policeman, postman etc. which was enormous fun – all un peu zig zag. My French was particularly fluent which baffled the butcher, for when I breakfasted with him this morning my vocabulary could do no more than 'Très bon café m'sieur'. I think he thought I was somebody else. We faire la chasse with them next Sunday which should be hilarious and fearfully dangerous. 'Yes my son I was severely wounded in the North African Campaign by a pissy postman who aimed at a wild pig.' I'll tell you about it next week. Announced today on the B.B.C. that the King is here – how splendid – but not you notice till Winston had done it first. I hope we see him. Saw a Bosche plane caught in our searchlights and shot down two nights ago – a wonderful sight, so clever it baffles me.

I tried to organise a dance for the troops – but the Mayor said 'No, we do not dance till France is free.' So I'm going to suggest a fête for the children – egg and spoon and three legged races – good for the entente and will help me to get eggs and maybe a pig. Sweet kids here, lots of baby girls. Heard from mine this week – Loo full of affection – Prudie complaining they never received the oranges 'But thanks all the same.' Her effort after the Victory was perfect: 'P.S. Awfully glad about Africa'. God how it restored one's sense of perspective. What is Armageddon compared with the Easter Holidays? I love you my darling beyond all reason.
Tam

Margaret to Tam — Halfway Cottage, 18 June 1943

My Beloved,

Your letter dated June 9th arrived this morning. You had your black curtain of depression wrapped tightly round your silly old head and shoulders. Oh my love don't be miserable, soon soon we shall be together again and you'll never have to be away from us again. Keep remembering how much I love you darling and that whatever happens you did the right thing. Full moon tonight, you make it 50, I 48. But suppose you are right. Have sent you a message and Johnny says you'll get it for our anniversary. Here we go round again for the fourth time. I don't know about you having taken the best years of my life, but you *gave* them to me. This I do know my love. We must meet *once* in every year we are married to each other, so I'll see you sometime this year!

Suppose you are now in your new place, hope you are comfort-

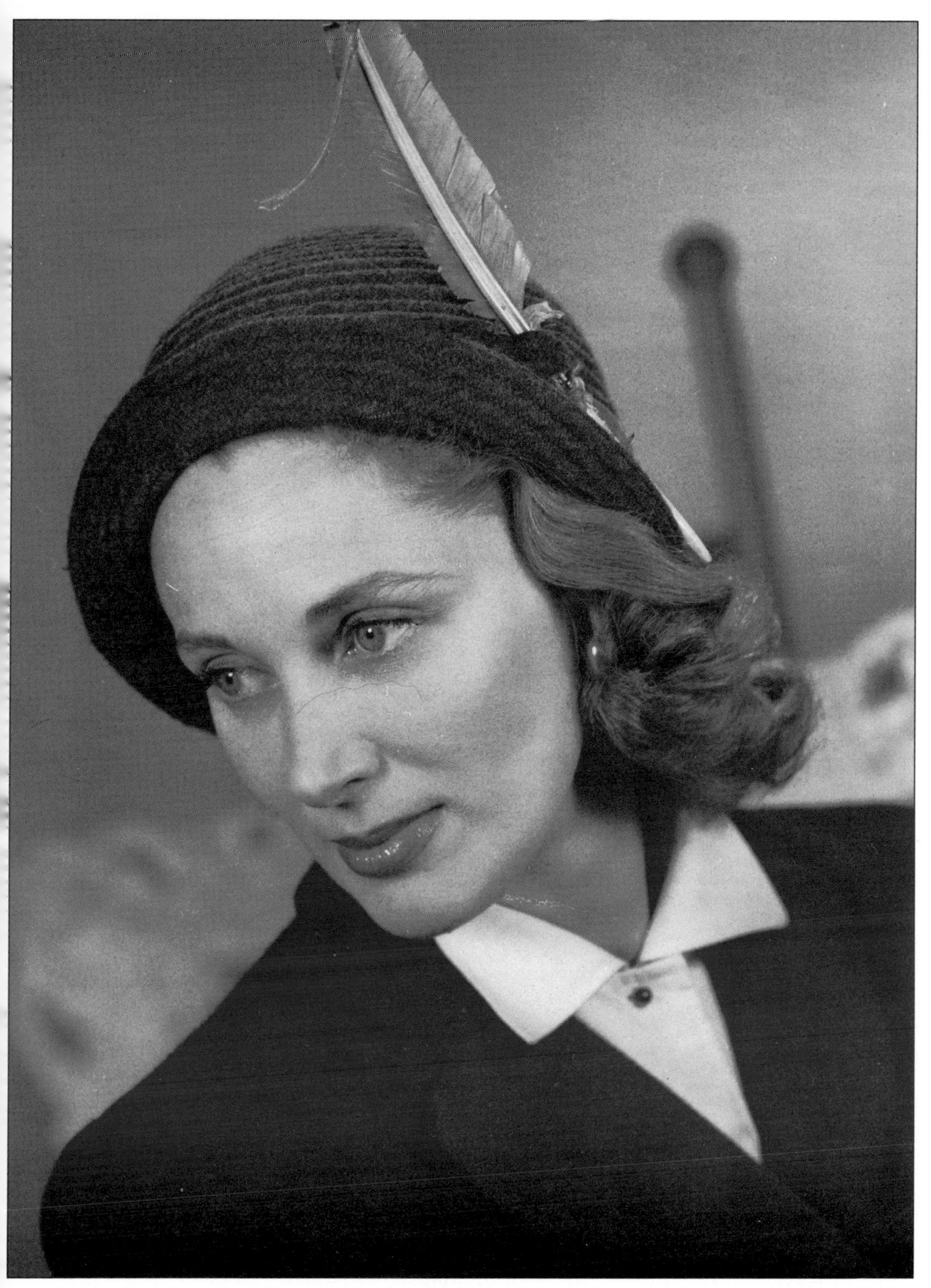

1. 'Australia's Premier Ambassadress of Beauty': Margaret in a war-time fashion shot.

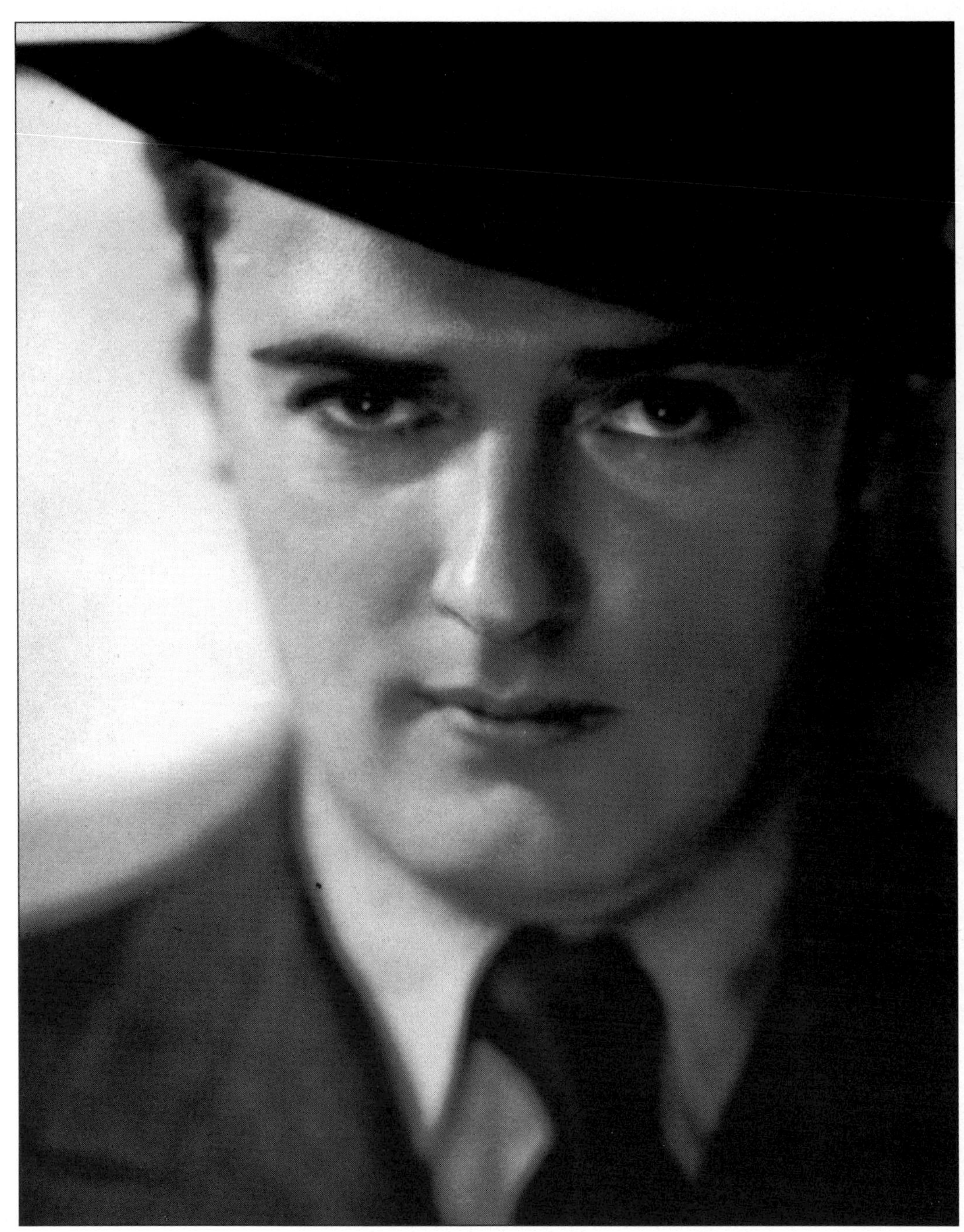

2. Tam in a still from the film *Rome Express* , 1932

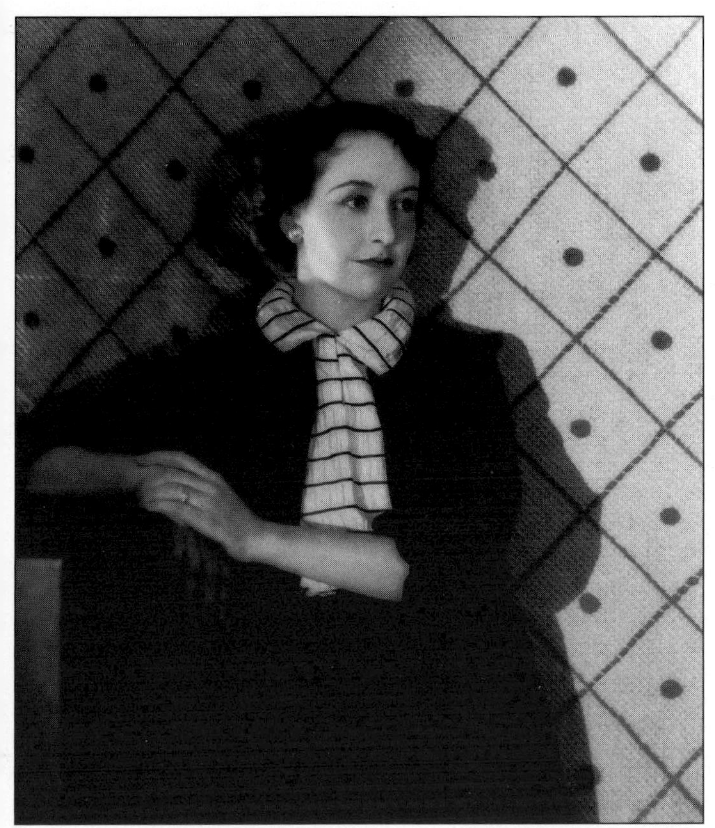

3. Gwynne Whitby, Tam's first wife, *c.* 1933. Margaret: 'I really do like Gwynne, she seems so honest and easy to talk to… she looked very young and very pretty.'

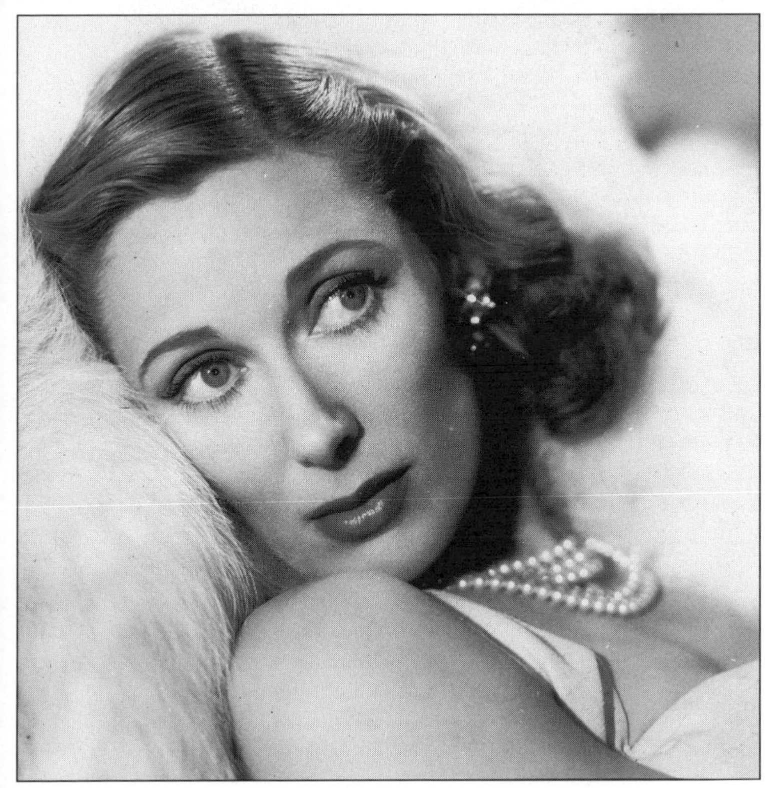

4. A pre-war publicity shot of Margaret

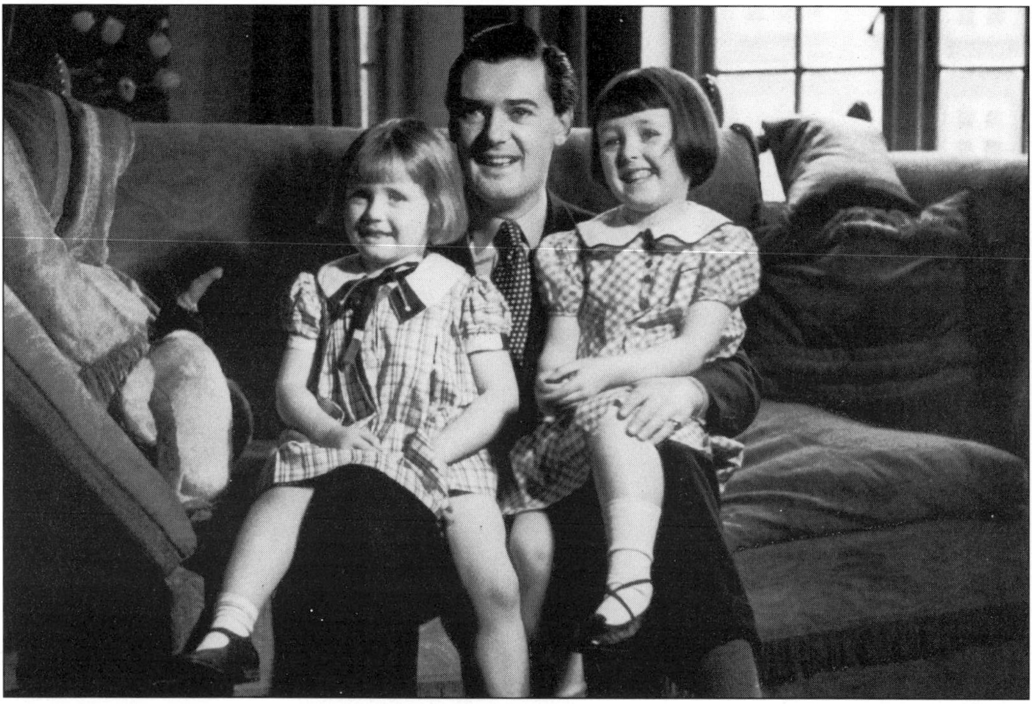

5. Tam with his daughters Loo (*right*) and Prue in the north London flat where they lived with Gwynne, their mother, *c.* 1937

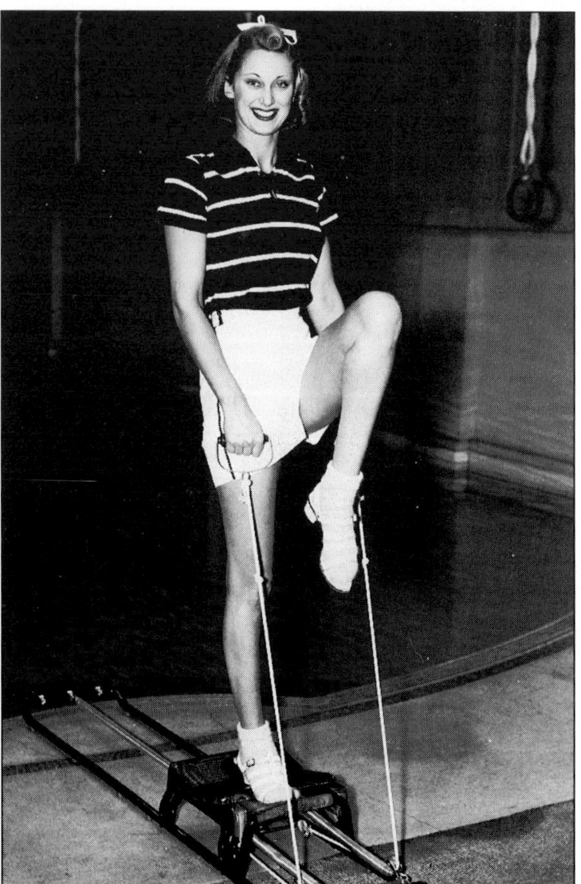

6. Margaret in a publicity shot taken during the 1938 filming of *Sailing Along*, directed by Sonnie Hale.

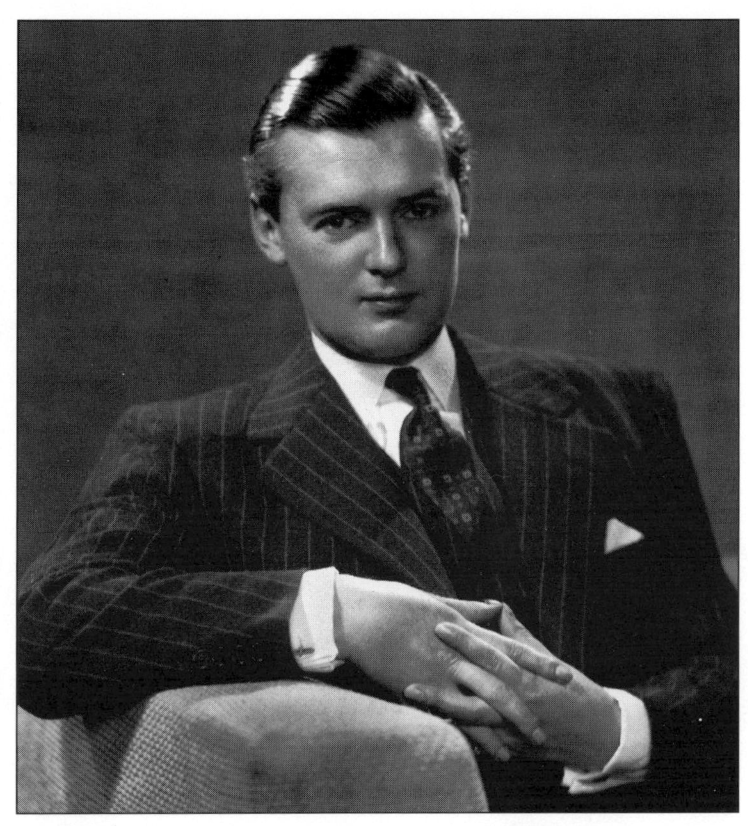

7. Tam in what he called Dorothy Wilding's 'flattering picture' of 1939

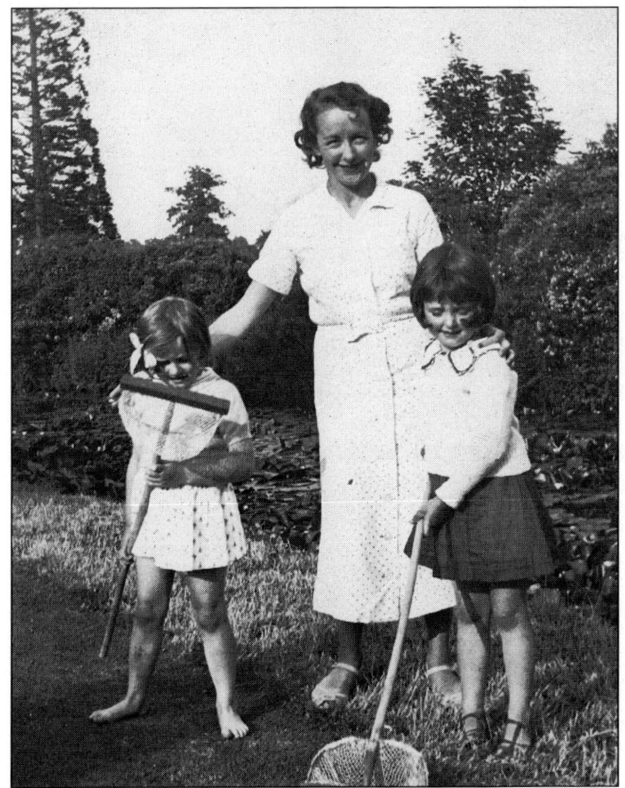

8. Gwynne with Loo (*right*) and Prue on the Isle of Wight, 1939

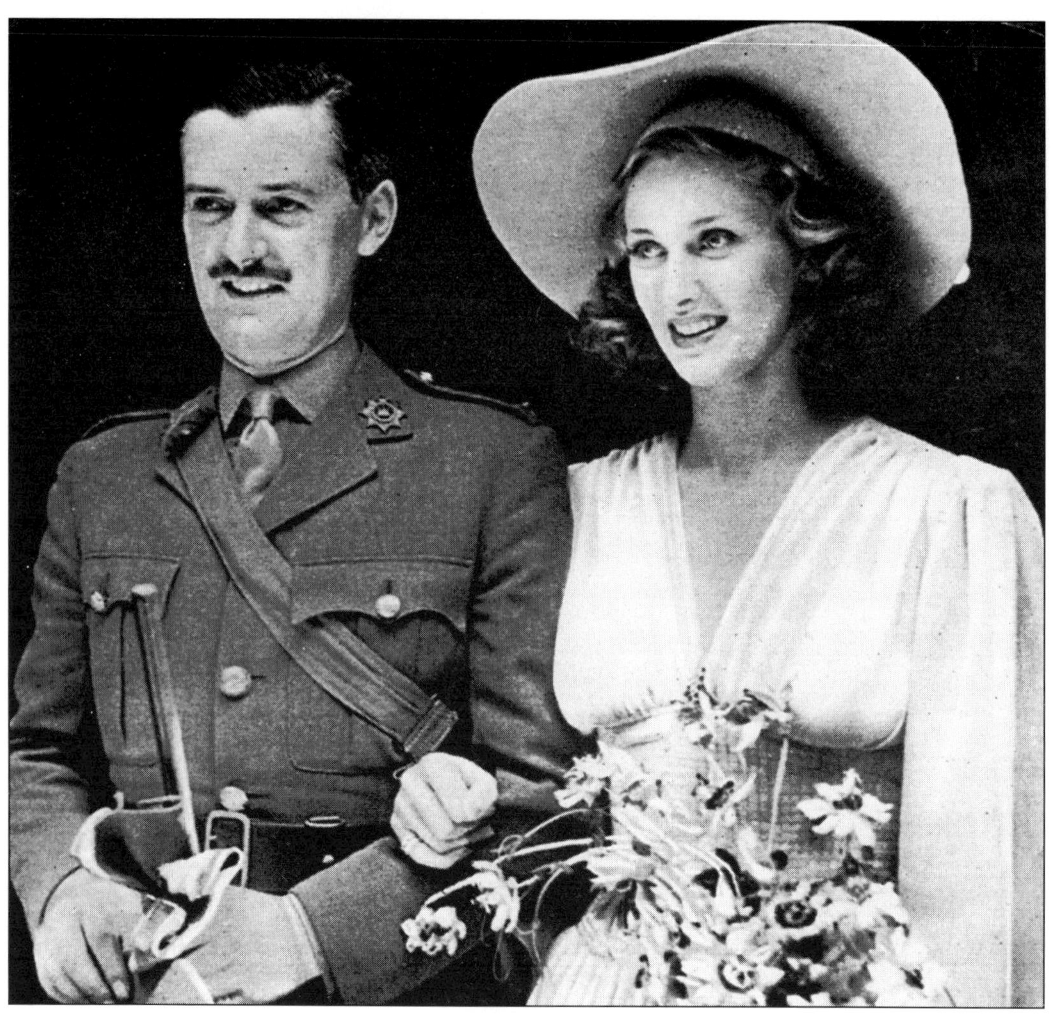

9. Tam and Margaret's wedding day, 21 June 1940. Margaret later wrote: 'Oh dear, that photograph made me very sad. It was such a desperate time for England and France but so glorious for Hugh and Margaret.'

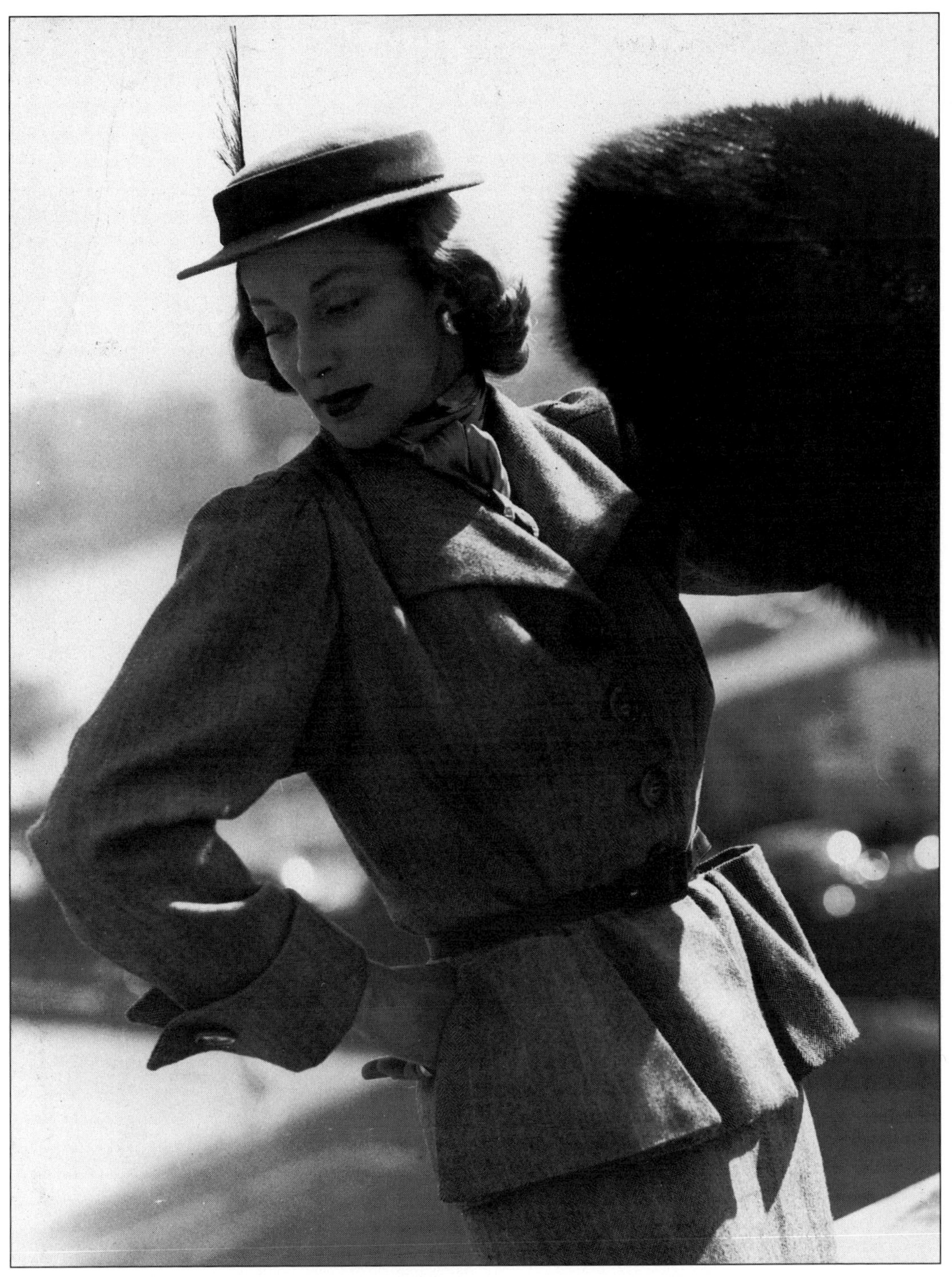

10. Margaret on a modelling assignment, probably in July 1940.
Tam was not enthusiastic about her having to work:
'I hate you doing those bloody photographs. I hate it.'

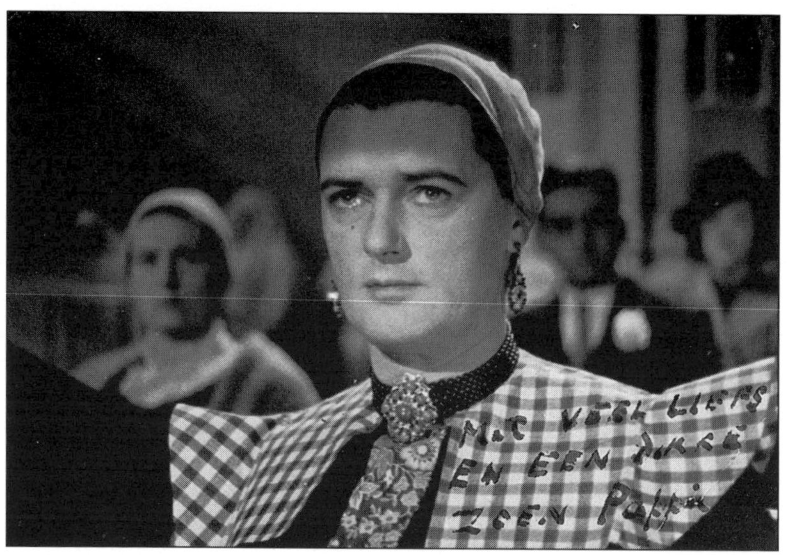

11. Tam disguised as a Dutch woman in the 1942 film *One of Our Aircraft is Missing* in which he played Frank Shelley. The inscription, written in Dutch, reads 'With much love and a big kiss from Daddy'.

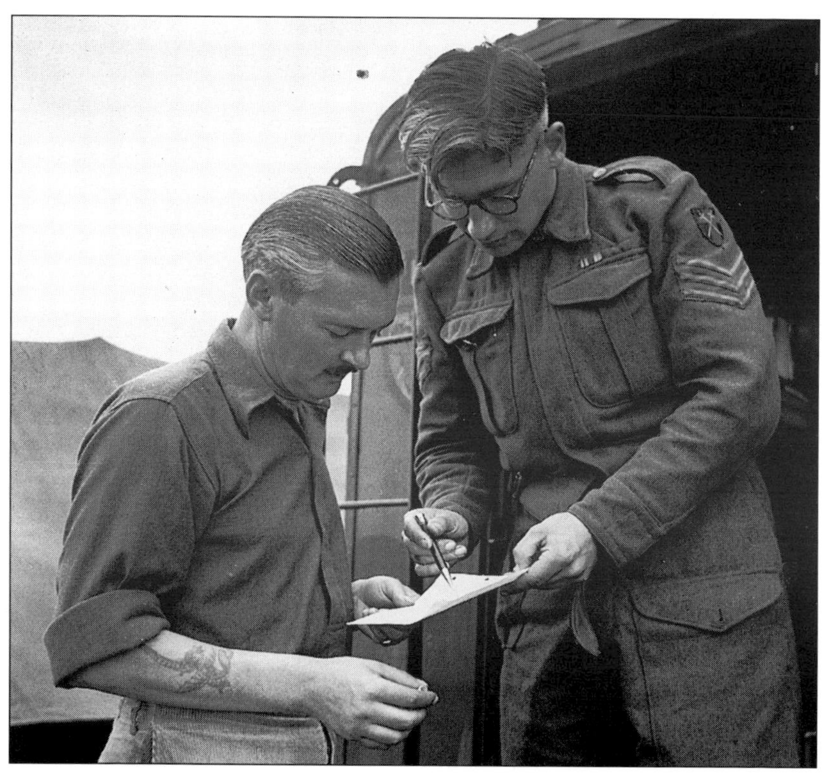

12. Captain H.A.G. Williams, Phantom Regiment (*left*), Tam's other self, here discussing the contents of a message from 21 Army group (undated).

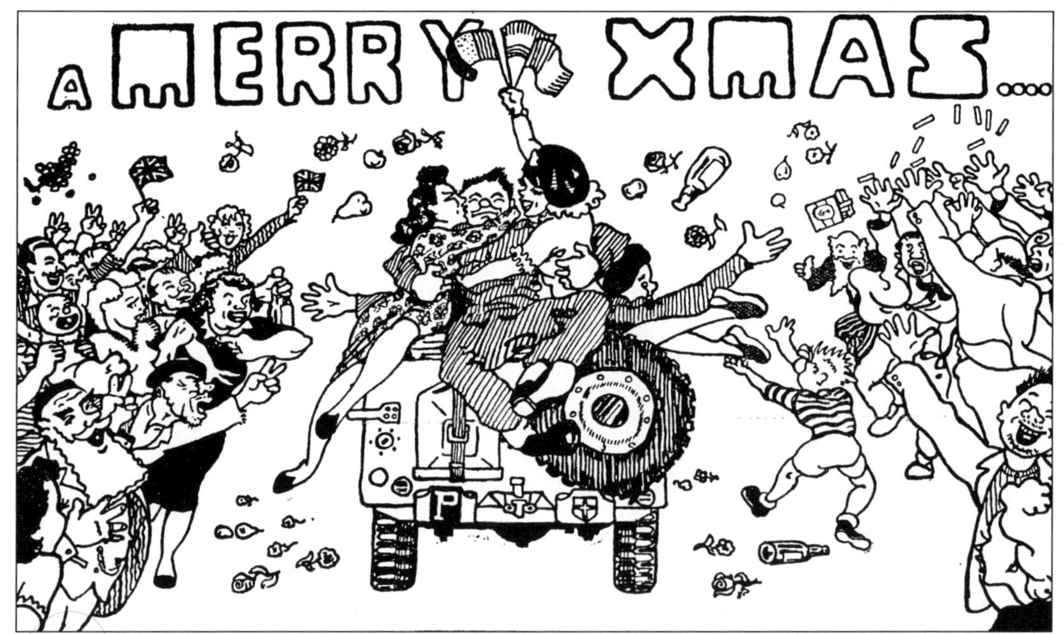

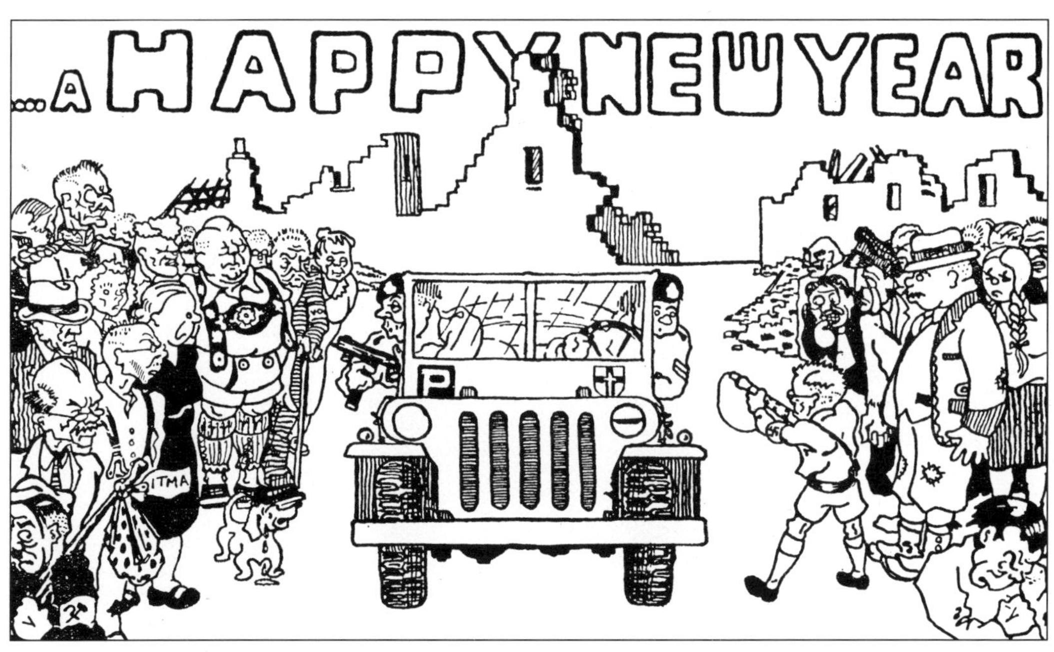

13. Phantom Christmas card, 1944. Tam: '…this one really is the last, next year we'll be together, to do Hugo's stocking and put up the holly and split a bottle in the process and share his onslaught at first light upon our hangovers.'

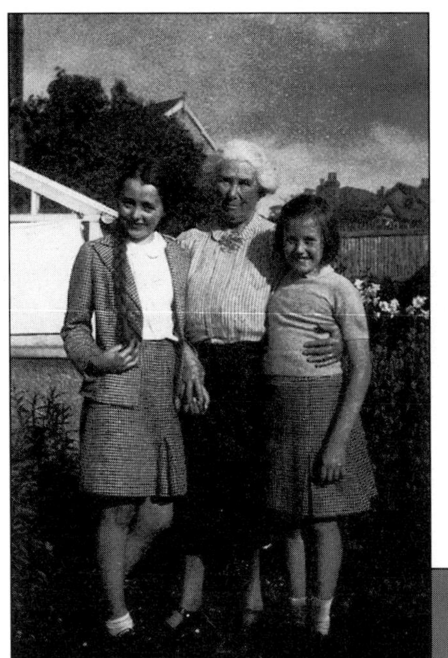

14. Tam's mother, 'my sweet old devil Silver', with Loo (*left*) and Prue, outside their digs in Cheltenham, 1943

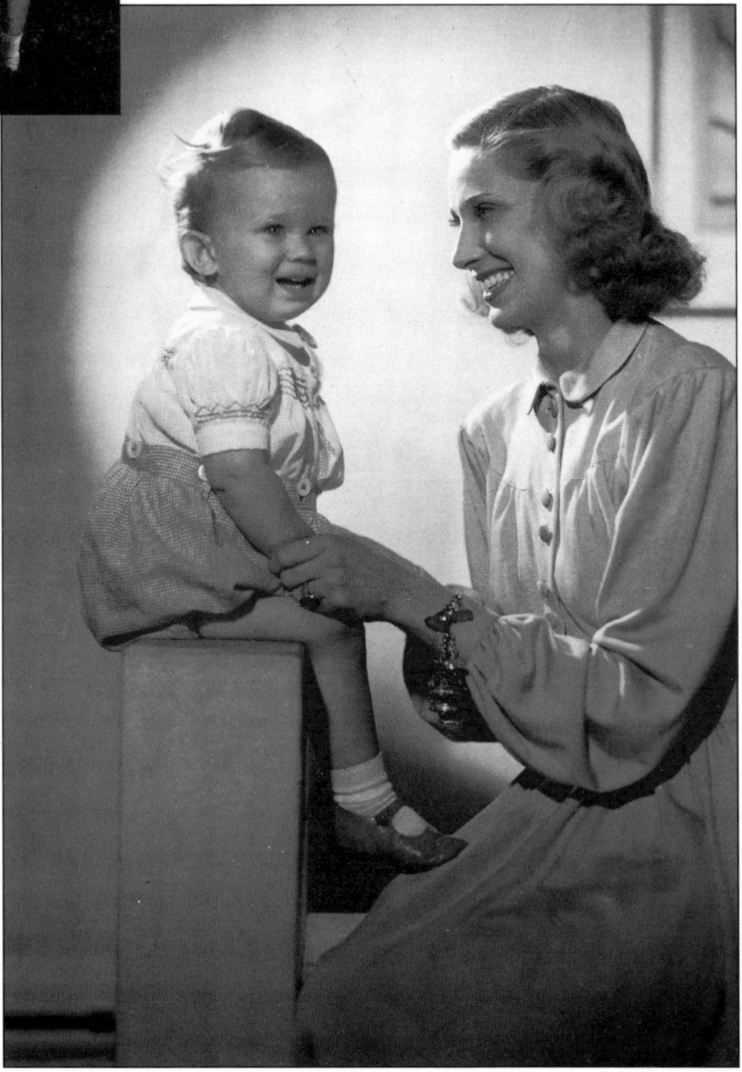

15. Margaret and Hugo *c.* 1944. 'How's my Hugo, I think of you both so much my darlings – apart from loving you I am so very proud of you.'

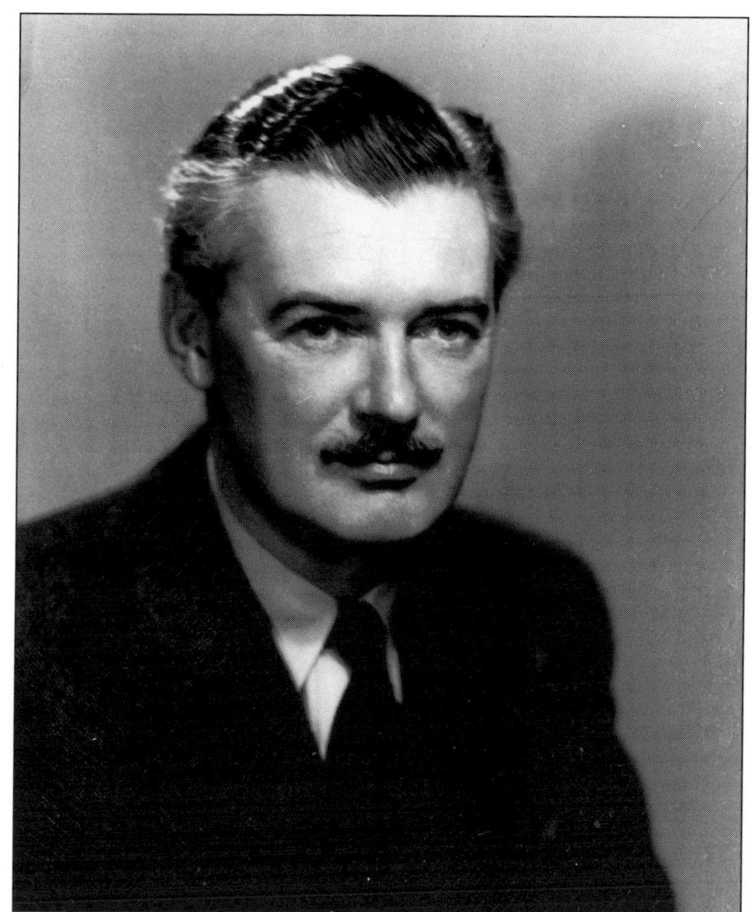

16. A post-war photograph of Tam, taken around January 1950. As early as August 1943 he was worried that he was ageing: 'Had a good look at my face this morning. It's a lot thinner and rather weary looking and I shall be as white as ermine before long.'

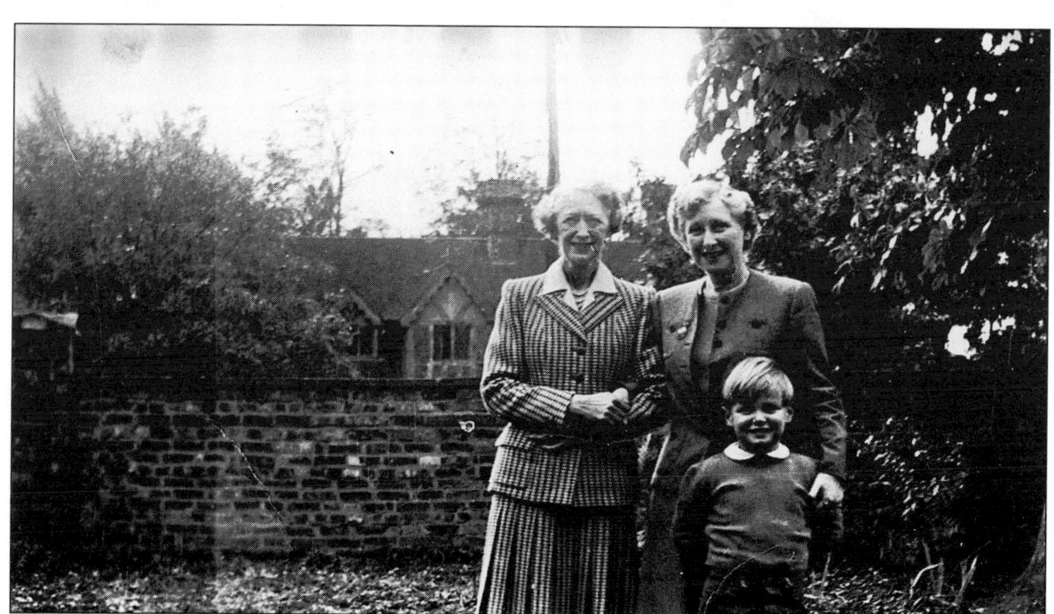

17. Margaret's mother Ruby (*left*) with her sister Phyllis and Tam and Margaret's second son Simon (born 1946) at Dorney, *c.* 1950

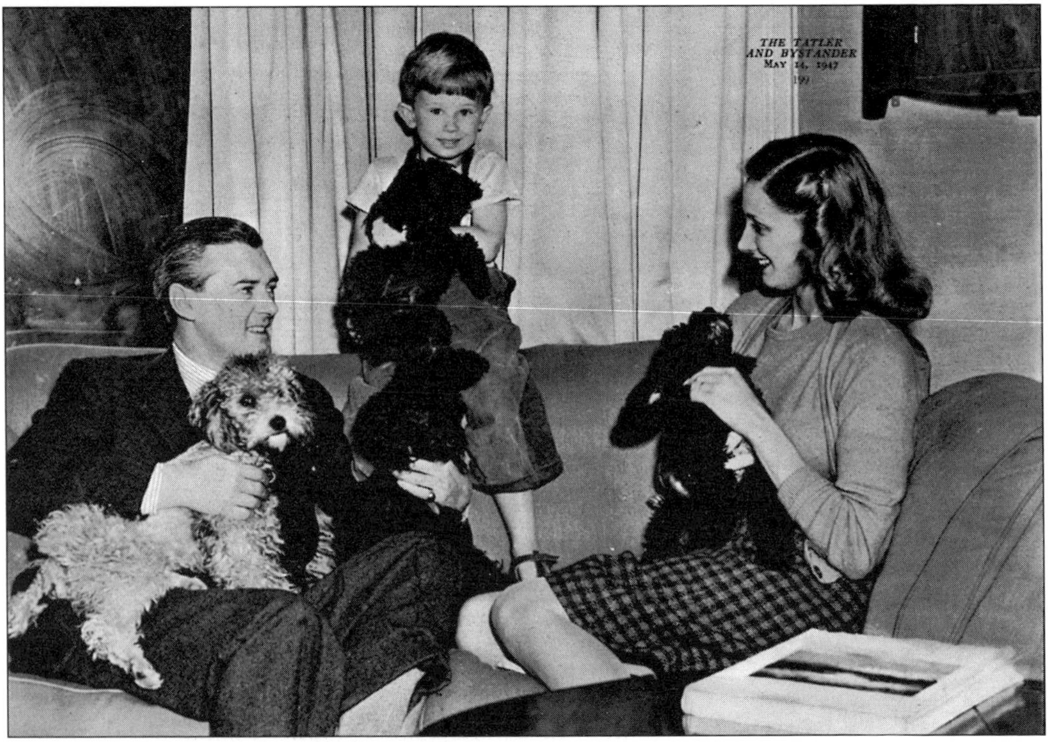

THE TATLER
AND BYSTANDER
MAY 14, 1947
199

18. 'The well-known group, Mum, Dad, the Brat and the Dogs. Suitable for Grand Pianos and insertion in the Tatler.' Tam, Margaret and Hugo, 1947

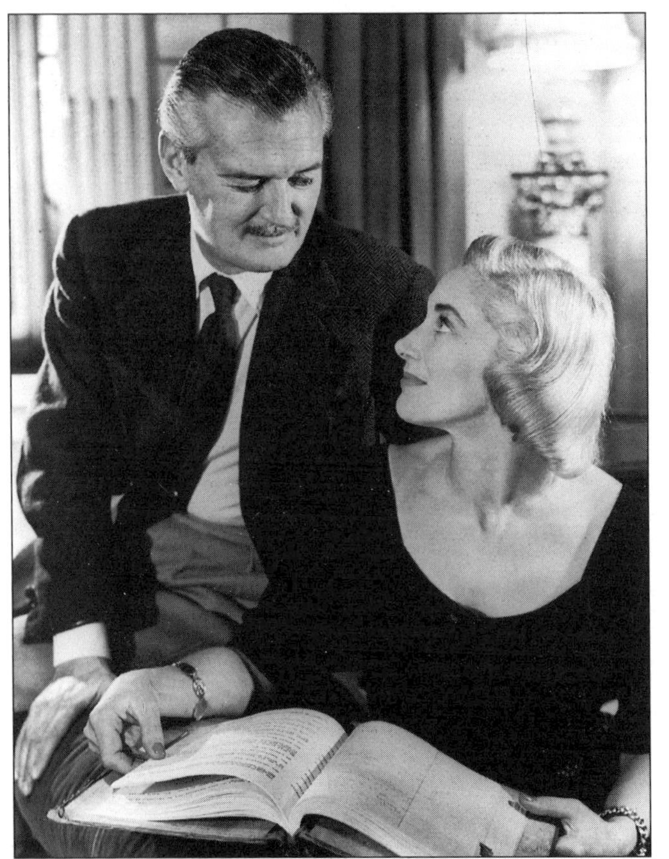

19. Tam and Margaret in the late 1950s, with the script of their play, *The Grass is Greener.*

able and can still swim. Have you seen the King yet? Now do take care of yourself my love and let me know if you want anything. I shall go to bed now and cuddle your old dressing gown. God bless you always, your M.

Tam to Margaret North Africa, 19 June 1943

Saw His Majesty the day before yesterday – we lined the route. He looked very smart and very brown and very young and although we waited a long time in the boiling sun I was glad I was there. In peace time it would have been Ascot Gold Cup Day and I should have seen him through my glasses driving up the course – my gray top hat held high. Strange contrasts but I'm used to them. Only about three or four of our Officers turned out which I thought was very rude – damn it he'd come a long way to see us all and the very least we could do was to go and shout a cheer.

You'll be reading soon maybe of activities in this theatre – I'm not concerned in them so don't worry or make the drama, later maybe. Say nothing to anyone. I only tell you so you won't get windy. I enclose a small gambling cheque. I've heard of a thing called a submarine suit, Austin Reeds, Regent St, ask for the manager. They're wonderfully warm and if you get wet they keep you afloat, and you can eat the lining. I believe if you can get one it will just keep me from freezing up. My darling this letter is disjointed and not saying what it should, for I'm writing against time and light. But what it should bring to you is my love my pretty – great gushing overpowering enormous waves of it and hope and optimism and the certain feeling that we're entering the last phase – I'm sure of it, a year no more. I adore you my darling, for always and always,

Tam

Margaret to Tam Halfway Cottage, 26 June 1943

Darling, darling, darling,

No news from you all week then Johnny rang to say that he had a letter from you for me and would bring it over. He came in about tea time and brought your letter and news that you were well and fairly happy in the new place,[1] which I do know the name of but had better not mention. However it is some small comfort to look at a map and know exactly where you are. Glad to hear what you told me in your letter but had gathered as much from Johnny. Sounds as if you are eating well my love, how about drinks?

Two days ago I had the last two messages I'd sent off for you returned with a note saying only very important messages could go through now, and then only through the Welfare Officer. I was miserable because the last one was for our anniversary saying – Remember three years ago darling – and I'd bunged it off in plenty of time in the hopes of it reaching you for the day. So all day went by and you had no message from me, but I suppose you knew what had happened my darling.

So glad you saw the King darling, pity so few of you turned out for him. I think he is magnificent. He got back home today thank God and bless his heart.

God bless you, all my love ALWAYS, your M.

1. Prior to the Allied invasion of Sicily Phantom was involved in training exercises in both Aqaba and Suez. Tam could have been at either.

Tam to Margaret North Africa, 2 July 1943

And Oh, my darling, a really magnificent mail. An airmail and two long letters from you, two from mother and a joint one from the girls. For more than an hour I was transported from this forest of cork trees, but am now back again alack and alas, in the middle of a four day scheme – our first since the battle – and it's rather like playing a poorly written love scene at an empty matinée with someone you've just slept the night with. One of my Coders was more succinct. 'Ain't this bloody deadly Sir?' His Majesty is ill advised. Medals should be given for exercises not campaigns. One would have the Bumper ribbon with the Bulldog or Spartan Star – 'For needless discomfort in the face of overwhelming boredom.' They must needs alter the procedure of the code and we're heading happily for a shambles. The Mayor of the village, who dined us the other evening, is a dentist and we have difficulty with the wireless when the old sod uses his electric drill! I find farce always so very near at hand in Phantom.

My dear girl I really must disabuse your mind about this quite fictitious report that I have been in any way a success. I floundered through the campaign as best I could – a military half-wit with no training in the particular job. It doesn't make any sort of sense and I beg you no more of it.

I've realised now that the secret of an enjoyable war is to be

where the spotlight is. One was exhilarated in the Summer of 1940 digging away at the Bexhill Grandstand, and so it is here. The rest has been so abysmally boring that it is just as impossible to describe as the excitement one had in the last days of the Tunis battle, or the feeling in the air now. But all the wonderful moments conjured by the imagination, like leading in the Derby winner or acknowledging thunderous applause as actor-author at the Haymarket, or writing a verse that was more than a rhyme, seem like mundane trivialities when one thinks of the moment when the door will open and you will be standing there.
Always, Tam

Tam to Margaret North Africa, 8 July 1943

Oh my darling I miss you so much – the sea and the sun and the brown rocks remind me unmercifully of you.

I want you, if you possibly can, to go down to Cheltenham. I'm worried about rooms for Mother next Winter. I've made this great point of the children staying on there and the only remaining snag is her comfort and welfare, for if she cracks up then they'll most certainly have to leave. She simply cannot do housemaid's work any more, if it means paying more then we'll have to pay more. Will you write and show concern and if necessary go down? If we can get through this winter we'll be home and dry.

I've had rather ill fortune with my dicing. You remember I won 4000 Frs, I've now taken a tinsy winsy tumble and have had to write a bunch of cheques amounting to £35. It should be in the bank alright, but I wanted it for you. Fuck. Sorry.

Had one of the most alarming and amusing nights of all time last night. The Hotel here has opened up an Officer's rest place and the Boule Table has been dug up from the cellar – you can guess the rest. Nobody to run the thing so Hugh Fraser and I seized what we thought was our big chance. We borrowed all the available ready we could and started crouping like crazy. Fate was unkind and a little over an hour later after we'd started we got smacked for 8000 frs. in one coup. There was a very ugly few minutes for we couldn't pay. I.O.U.'s were hastily written and Robin Baring[1] was dispatched to the Camp to fetch the profits of the men's Canteen, and with under a mille for capital we carried on. I was really terrified and Hugh was dead white and very sweaty – we had no idea how we could fix the Canteen money. Robin returned and we redeemed our I.O.U.'s, and then by the grace of

God the Navy arrived very determined to wipe us out. We recouped completely something like 11 mille and made about 800 each. Phantom was there in force very pissy and squealing with delight at our fearful danger – this morning there was a notice in the Mess. 'Until further notice Officers will not run the bank at Boule' – so we've arranged that the Grenadiers shall run it! Don't be cross with me. It was enormous fun and I've always hankered after crouping – but one needs champagne, not rather warm, still, sweet white stuff. I've had great remorse about the money I've lost and will be good from now on. I return by myself to Carthage next week but for how long I don't know. Anchor Detachment this time. I love you my beloved more than life and life I only love because of you. Hello Hugo. Always and always,
Tam

1. Captain R.W. Baring, Royal Artillery 12 Corps.

Margaret to Tam Bigbury-on-Sea, South Devon, 9 July 1943

My own most beloved,

I was a bit low and leaving Halfway Cottage was a bigger sentimental jolt than I thought it would be.[1] So many wonderful times we have had there and it is strange living in the tiny house which has no memories of you my love.

Oh well, it will all pass and the sun will shine and this will all seem like a nasty dream.

Look after yourself darling and stay in love with me and think of me.

Hugo sends love and kisses. Johnny says he's just written to you.
I'll love you till I die darling,
Always and always,
Your M.

1. Forced to leave Halfway Cottage when the lease expired, all Margaret could find to rent in Dorney was a smaller cottage called Two Gates. Between leaving one and moving into the other she went on holiday to Devon.

Tam to Margaret North Africa, 15 July 1943

Oh my Darling,

Forgive me my darling I am not hungover but still fearfully zig zag. I have breakfasted and am still atrocious. As you may have gathered I caught up with the Henson[1] crowd last night, and this morning I'm inclined to apply for a regular commission. How good of them all to come here – this I mean, really admirable. But having made the gesture, having decided and given their sacrifice, they might have rehearsed. All doing their old single acts. Bea[2] superb, Leslie pissed, no make up, no sparkle, no wit, no punch. The master of spontaneity the victim of staleness. And Miss Leigh[3] having travelled so far and so graciously, recited, but only very little and oh so poorly, a little bit from *Alice in Wonderland* and a cheap little verse about Plymouth. Thin, amateur, impertinent; without talent, charm or grace, but good enough for the troops. Christ I sweated with annoyance. If they'd worked only in the mornings for a week, they could have done something, but no. The whole thing was a display of carelessness and laziness. Afterwards I got very pissy with Leslie but held my peace. So that's why I spew it out on you, forgive me please my darling.

I shall write to you tomorrow and apologise for being so drunken. Good morning my darling and the same to Hugo, Tam

1. Leslie Henson (1891-1957), actor and producing manager, took a group of performers out to North Africa to entertain the troops.
2. Beatrice Lillie (1989-1989), Canadian actress.
3. Vivien Leigh (1913–67).

Tam to Margaret — North Africa, 18 July 1943

My Darling,

Still staying with Jack and taking things very steady – the moon is as round as a penny and so yellow it makes not a silver but a golden path across the sea and as usual I'm filled with a great surge of longing for you – oh my beloved I love you and miss you and want you so appallingly. Fearfully hot and the flies are ghastly. Never less than half a score on one's hands and arms, and one is continually making ridiculous little movements to dislodge them. How lovely when flies means something one adjusts before leaving once more.

I shall want snaps of my son's reaction to the sea and his first mouthful of sand – it says a lot for my character, and for my love for you that I'm not a little jealous. He'll be so wonderful on the beach – a crab, a shell, a limpet, seaweed, castles and canals and pools, and the great insoluble mystery of the tide going in and out, and never quite being in the same place as you were the morning before, the misery of lunchtime and the ecstatic joy of after breakfast. You must remember it all for me. And remember this for me too. Nanny and Hugo don't need a holiday – you do so take it.

Good, great news from Russia and not too bad from Sicily.[1] Have so much to tell you, if only we had a fire and a bottle – but if we had a fire and a bottle all I should want would be cushions on the floor and lovely records. Sometimes I can't imagine it. On the other hand sometimes I imagine it quite delightfully. I use the idiom 'on the other hand' deliberately. If the mails are haywire don't worry I am as constant as the night and day. God bless my love to you for always and always,
Tam

1. On 13 July 1943 the Germans were routed in a tank battle at Kursk and the Allies captured Augusta and Ragusa on the island of Sicily.

Tam to Margaret North Africa, 22 July 1943

My darling,

God it's been hot. Drinking water becomes as warm as the normal bath, one is permanently sweating, utterly exhausted, fly-blown, weak and ill-tempered. One's had Algerian wine. Maybe if we fight on we shall one day arrive in a country where there's something fit to drink. How pleasant to be advancing through the Côte d'Or with one's water bottle filled with Pouilly. After the war we'll make a little tour in search of food and drink, and all day long we'll laze and make love on the banks of the Loire, and in the evening, carefully and quietly and with diligence we'll become superbly and serenely drunk. I suppose we shan't though. Hugo will want to be taken to Frinton for the tennis tournament. We shall have to conceal all knowledge of snow from him – it would be dreadful if he developed a Winter Sport habit.

The war seems to be going really well – surely next year will finish it – Europe anyway. But I'm not sure I agree with bombing Rome.[1] You only have to drop one down the Pope's chimney and you've split the world in two.

Rest yourself in Devon and take things really steady. My love to all of them and to you my Margaret,
Always and always,
Tam

1. On 19 July five hundred American bombers dropped one thousand tons of high explosive on Rome, remarkably avoiding all the historical sites. Eight days later Italy was suing for peace.

Tam to Margaret North Africa, 28 July 1943

My darling,

I got your letter and snaps of Hugo and pictures of you in *The Lamp Still Burns*. Thank you my beloved and you're very pretty – so is Granger's[1] hair-do. Very anxious to hear news of the opening, sounds suspiciously as though you've made a success. Well done.

I imagine at the moment you're having hideous moving trouble. I wish I were there to get in the way. Depressed and disappointed, I was all set to go with E Squadron to Sicily, but now it's all been cancelled and I'm back with K Squadron on the mountain top with no job in sight except to organise a rest camp! Can't help feeling that this is now a backwater for I'm convinced Italy will retire hurt as soon as she possibly can. Mussolini has really made himself ludicrous. There's nothing so contemptible as a silly villain – to be hated and laughed at. The two worst achievements in life, for then there can be no pity. I suspect strongly that we're in the process of double crossing and double dealing. For two years Russia has groaned for a second front – a Western front. Now you mark my words, nothing will happen till next year, then we shall have a go, deliver the coup de grace – victory, honour, glory, well done England and America, and instead of us it will have been Russia who was the second front. It's the bloody cock house spirit again and you can trace it right down from that level to Phantom Squadrons and the Devonshire regiment. Monstrous. Surely to God we could mount an invasion from England this Autumn and give Russia a chance to bang in the winter.[2] I can't bear to think that we're not quite honourable – if we're not you might just as well scratch the word out of the dictionary for nobody else is. Maybe these thoughts are due to the fact that we've been shrouded in cloud for forty-eight hours, or maybe it's boredom.

If the devil crept into my tent tonight and offered me a week with you in exchange for a year of my life, or even my immortal soul, I'd close the deal in a flash. By the time you get this you'll be in Devon, watching our son finding shells and little crabs and wondering why sand looks so delicious and tastes disgusting, and why the sea makes such a noise. Oh lucky woman. Write and tell me that you're fond of me and miss me and want me with you – I seldom think of anything but the end of it all – me and three or four million other people – dear God

to be free again. We'll sleep all day and sing all night out of sheer joy.
Always my beloved,
Tam

1. Stewart ('Jimmy') Granger (1913–93), film actor.
2. The Allies could not mount an invasion of France until the Mediterranean sector was closed and troops fighting there released for duty elsewhere.

Tam to Margaret North Africa, 4 August 1943

My darling Margot,

Have a most appalling cold and I've blown a little blood vessel, so every time I blow my nose the damn thing bleeds which results in continual sniffing. Broke another one on the tip of my elbow, which is the size of a lemon and the colour of a plum – arm quite useless at the moment, which means I can only wash one armpit. It's produced Tennis Elbow. Can you beat that for a battle scar! I shall call it Tunis Elbow. But really I've never felt such a fool.

Soon it will be six months since we said goodbye – that surely must be at least a third of the time of the separation. And a third is nearly half way. It may be worse for us when we're apart, which after all is only fair, for it's much more wonderful when we're together than for anybody else in the world. Start seven days leave on Saturday. Leave. An empty word unless it means you. Mum keeps saying in her letters how she loves your letters and is so fond of you. Think the idea of Ruby going there for the winter is *simply bristling with danger*. You know I never underline unless it's something – well something. Don't you agree? Darling your letters are wonderful about Hugo – I can follow his growing and developing beautifully, and although it fills me with envy, and makes my heart very heavy, I'm so grateful to you my sweet. I love and adore you for always and always,
Tam

Tam to Margaret North Africa, 10 August 1943

My Darling,

Am on leave at the moment and my great news is – I've had a bath – a hot bath yesterday. March 22nd – to August 9th. God it was heaven. I used that lovely soap you sent me. I managed to get a room in a local Hotel which is run as an Officers' rest place. A balcony with a lovely view, and it's fun having a mirror and a proper basin. Had a good look at my face this morning, it's a lot thinner and rather weary looking and I shall be as white as ermine before long, so I call it more than sweet and sympathetic of you to be following me. I think of you and Hugo playing in Devon and my heart nearly jumps the distance that separates us.

In a letter or two ago you said John[1] had said he'd like to paint you. Wonderful. But I've always heard that with him the words paint and poke are synonymous so follow it up but take care my pretty, for I'll cut his beard off, if on my return, I find you've been a fool. Can't think of anything in the world I'd like more than a really lovely picture of you. Nice for Hugo too when we're together in the Church yard. I so often wonder how much longer we have together. Six years already – under hard and difficult conditions and bloody separations – it makes me hope we both live to be very old to make up for it. I love you very much my darling – more than distance and more than time can alter, so if the war goes on for twenty years and letters never reach me and I have no news, I shall find you somehow and begin where we left off, which as far as I remember was with a bottle of the dear stuff,

Always,
Tam

1. Augustus John (1878–1961), British painter.

Margaret to Tam — Two Gates, Dorney, near Windsor
17 August 1943

Oh my darling,

What a strange, lonely, disturbed feeling it gave me to read your letter this morning dated only 7 days ago and to know that you were on leave and but for this fucking war and our separation we'd have been together. And to know that you were on leave at the same time as I was in Devon fancying myself on holiday, ye blue Gods!!

Then just after I'd read your letter Tony Warre rang. Sweet!! I'm going over to lunch with them tomorrow. Golly, golly how I shall eat up his news of you. You said your face was thinner and that you looked weary and your hair is much whiter – darling what could be more attractive? I'd wait until the day I died to see such a person with such a face. And I worship you too my best beloved forever. Wish I'd been at that bath with you though.

Goodnight my adored one.
Always your own M.

Tam to Margaret North Africa, 20 August 1943

Next week we should know our fate. I have a horrible feeling it may be Persia, why I can't imagine. News still spendid. But I wish Sicily would pack up – if she doesn't by the end of September I lose a fiver to Springett.[1] There's a little Italian prisoner doing tailoring at the hospital up here who had seen me on the screen – dubbed in Italian – who was very puzzled when he discovered I couldn't speak a word. I got a French interpreter to explain to him but even then he wasn't convinced. I fear this letter is about nothing, but life is as empty as my bottle of whisky will be by bedtime so forgive me if it's dull. Yours never are. But to finish here's this for you:–

I am a man of impeccable taste
In all matters concerning the choice
Of the beauty, the charm and the grace of a girl
And the gentleness of her voice
Did I not choose Margaret?

I am a man whom fortune favours
And God smiles upon from above
I am a man unlucky at cards
But undoubtedly lucky in love,
Did I not win Margaret?

I am a man who is clever indeed
I am both shrewd and astute
I am a man of wisdom and wit
Oh, I am most certainly vute[2]
Did I not wed Margaret?

Much love always,
Tam

1. Given the strength of the Allied forces – 150,000 troops landed on 10 July, protected by 1,000 aircraft, and over half a million men were put ashore before the campaign was over – Sicily took a long time to capture. She finally fell when Messina was taken on 17 August.
2. This may have been a private word of Tam and Margaret's, the meaning of which is now lost.

Margaret to Tam Two Gates, Monday 23 August 1943

My own Tamèd Darling,

Letter from you this morning, dated Aug 15th, not bad, eh? You sound rather depressed and low sweetheart and I don't suppose getting a letter from me saying I was a bit creaky has helped. I always feel that I can cope and as long as I think that way all will be well.

Last Wed I went over to Richmond to lunch with Tony Warre. He met me at the station in a very insecure pony trap and off we went. He started to chat about you and all the world in general almost immediately and behaved with me as if he's known me for ages and only seen me yesterday. I *really* liked him. Unfortunately his wife Arbel was away working, but actually I suppose he talked more and told me more being alone. He got maps and charts out and went through the whole thing with me. Bless him I loved it all. He gave me a picture of you in a group and made me feel he was very fond of you indeed. Anyway I enjoyed my day and came home happier than I've been for ages. Being near someone who'd seen you recently, I suppose.

Am enclosing some snaps of our boy in this letter. He looks very plain I know but he really is very sweet to look at and his colouring is lovely now. Blue eyes, hair the colour of a new penny and rather streaky, and his brown skin. I suppose you'll have got the other snaps I sent which were taken by Niven, and the tiny piece of his hair. I wonder you've not mentioned it. Let me know.

Shall see Silver in London tomorrow. Poor old girl sounds exhausted and terribly fed up with life. Hope to be able to cheer her up a bit.

God bless, watch over and take care of you my most beloved, I'm always with you, yours always in fact,
And I love you too,
Always your M.

Tam to Margaret North Africa, 28 August 1943

My beloved,

Had a curt and uncourteous letter from the Income Tax asking for some quite ridiculous sum. Write and say I'm unlikely to be traceable till after the war. Do you ever realise the enormous amount of money we've got to make after the war? But I have plans. Just been reading Jane's *Persuasion*, not quite so perfect as *Pride and Prejudice*, but pure joy all the same. And anyway, away away from Twentieth Century chaos and the North African glare, into the quiet of fashionable Bath. The heroine so very sweet and the hero as full of pride as ever. I think it might dramatise. Did some Shakespeare at the hospital concert the other evening and was as nervous as a cat. God knows what a London first night will be like with all the knockers [critics] waiting and hoping. I doubt if I'll make it. Sometimes I really do doubt it. I wonder if I'd run screaming from the theatre just as they called the quarter.[1] Oh dear how frightful it will be. Four years next Tuesday since I was in the theatre. Four years, which but for you I don't think I could have borne. We're so bored here now it's ghastly – people have started growing and shaving off moustaches – a certain sign of utter decay. News still wonderful. D'you realise we've had no bad news for over six months? If we invaded now the war would be over this year – even so I think not much more than nine or ten months. I adore you my lovely lovely Margaret, and I always and always shall. Tam

1. The 'quarter' is the call given to actors twenty minutes before curtain-up.

Margaret to Tam — Two Gates, 31 August 1943

Lovely sunny day and I've had a letter from you and a telegram from Dick Springett saying he has seen you and that you are in 'great heart'. So I'm feeling on top of the world. Your letter dated 27th says that a move for you is on the tapes[1], a lovely time of year darling for that part of the world. But it somehow seems so much further away. However you sound quite pleased about it so all is well. Good luck and take care of yourself. Oh darling you sound so really optimistic, do you really think it will all be so soon? I do agree with you about the slow crumble, for who is there to make an armistice with? Certainly not Hitler. Slovakia now in revolt so she is next, and then Hungary and so eventually the lot![2] It is really all such a colossal crumble of, as you say, countries *not* cities that one feels unable to take it in. I do not, however, think it will be over as soon as you do darling. However you are in a better position than me to know. Unless you are too close to it. On the other hand the disintegration has gone too far perhaps. I just can't even guess any more. Shall I see you before the 70th moon do you think my darling?

I was thinking as I walked out with Hugo the other day what a truly lucky girl I am. After 7 years the man I love and want more than anyone else in the whole world loves and wants me too. Oh yes darling, let us be awfully careful how we spend our precious years together. Let us not be foolish and muck them up and give each other unnecessary worry or hurts. Let us just be happy and

help others to be happy too. Oh hark at me and my utopian ideas. I suppose we'll fight like cat and dog sometimes and be filthy to people we don't like. But just let us not forget these five years apart. I do love you my love, do take care,
Always your M.

1. With most of the 8th Army already in Sicily Tam could reasonably expect his unit to join them.
2. Mussolini's fall from power on 25 July and the consequent demise of Fascism in Italy, coupled with the rebellions in Slovakia and Hungary, must have made people feel that before long Germany would succumb to the same infection.

Margaret to Tam Two Gates, 2 September 1943

My own Tamèd Beloved,

Remember being in your dressing room 4 years ago tonight darling.[1] How all the old drunks came flocking for a drink and reassurance. Oh dear! How much drunker we'd have got if we'd known it was to last four years. Ye Gods what a slice out of the most important years of our lives. Such precious years my darling. But in a way, they've bound us together much more surely than anything else could have done. I'd never be able to live the years after the war with anyone but you ever. Do you know what I mean Darling? O Golly now that this is the end of the month I'm terribly anxious to know what you will do. So terribly anxious. Persia would be the end darling. God bless you darlingest one,
ALWAYS AND ALWAYS,
Your M.

1. It was the fourth anniversary of Britain's declaration of war on Germany.

Margaret to Tam Dorney, Sunday 5 September 1943

My Tam my darling, I wonder, oh how I wonder where you are now, still sitting in the corkforests or even perhaps on your way to our enchanted isle of Aug '39,[1] or wonder of wonders on your way to Dorney Common.[2]

Had what is known as 'One of those weekends'. Sat afternoon helped entertain 30 cadet officers of the St John's Ambulance Brigade and Sat night I went to the Aspro Factory to raffle Whisky Gin Port and 2 lemons for the P.O.W. fund.[3] Plenty of Whisky, plenty of food and everyone trying to be as nice as possible, but I was overcome with a longing to go home the moment I arrived and that was that. However, I got a nice little sum of money for their fund considering the types there, and everyone seemed fairly satisfied.

Persian Gulf is 100–8 at the moment and we are pledged for the sum of three each way. 0K? Hope you have a good reason for this darling. N. Africa is a long way from the racing world.

Darling you are in my thoughts all day. Our next Wedding Day you think. Oh dear, I wonder. In the meantime go on loving me darling and I'll wait here for you,
Always your own M.

1. Margaret is referring to a holiday they took in Capri.
2. In fact, Tam remained in North Africa until 11 September.
3. As a local celebrity Margaret was involved in several fund-raising ventures.

Tam to Margaret North Africa, 5 September 1943

My beloved,

You have been an angel about writing and dear God what a difference to the day when I hear from you. I think it's odds on our coming back, maybe not, maybe further away, but I think a couple of months and you'll be hearing the telephone. Anyway it's worth while getting excited about. Don't tell anyone yet there's a chance I may be returning until you hear definitely. Oh my darling Margaret, where shall we go, where eat, where sleep and make love and talk and giggle? I shall borrow some money for I must have you to myself – first in London and then maybe we'll go and catch a glimpse of the Autumn if we're in time. Shall we have another baby if I come back? It's just about the perfect separation – about two and a half years, and we could get it over with almost before the war was finished. A Peace baby by six or seven weeks I'd say. I don't quite know how you feel about it any more. Be good my sweet and lovely Margaret – wait for me. Wait for me. I don't think I shall be long.

Had a deadly exercise last week down on the plain – very hot and fly blown and the Goddam Arabs stole my lavatory seat. A kiss on the back of the boy's neck,
Always and always,
Tam

Tam to Margaret North Africa, 8 September 1943

Well my darling!

I couldn't be sorrier for my last letter. I boobed. I bogged it. I gave you to understand it was 9–4 on our coming home. Tonight I find I'm off as anchor to E Squadron. Naturally my first reaction was to get fearfully drunk. Where we go I can only guess. Personally I think Greece. Though the other popular opinion is Italy. Why? Anyway the news is splendid[1] and I reckon the European war will be over by my birthday.[2] *Don't worry* if you don't hear from me for a week or two.

Always and always,
Tam

1. The Allies landed on mainland Italy on the night of the 8/9 September and captured Reggio di Calabria, strategically vital to the 'toe' of Italy.
2. 6 March.

Tam to Margaret North Africa, 10 September 1943

I know the form a bit better now. Bella Italia. Even Chianti will be a change for the better. I'm through with vin rose for ever. Rumour all day long we've invaded France. If true I think Christmas will see it over. There's a general crumble going on. Am looking forward to this new job though, should be fearfully interesting, and as usual my love disgracefully safe. Hoping to get a sufficiency of pink gin en route.

Slept only one hour last night – the sweat trickling over my eyebrows into the sockets. Drinking water is quite hot enough to shave in with comfort. Hitler speaking tonight. What? Why? A blood and sweat and toil and tears one I wouldn't be surprised. Has any moment in the history of the world been quite so exciting? How terrible – how like a eunuch not to be a minute part of it. The flies can't even scare me out of it.

Love, love for ever and always,
Tam

Margaret to Tam Two Gates, 14 September 1943

Tamèd my Tamèd,

Your wonderful wonderful letter arrived today dated Sept 5th. Golly, if only it were true my love, if only. Yes, yes, yes you are quite right far better to tell me and let me be excited even if it is only for a little while with a disappointment after all. Where shall we go? What shall we do indeed? Why darling to Paradise if they will have us there. I could never meet you in a public place darling, it must be somewhere where we are all alone. I've so much to tell you and do to you and then one day I'll have a wonderful weep on your shoulder just for the misery of the time without you. Golly, how the news goes. But what is all this about the Germans rescuing Musso.[1] No confirmation from us so far but I suppose it is true. Bugger this pen and the ink and the paper, I think they do this sort of thing on purpose now to try to lessen the mails. I think the paper's a sort of April fool joke, don't you?

You need have no fear about Hugo not giving you a grand welcome darling. He still gives kisses to all your pictures and never makes the age old baby error of calling any man daddy. You are his man!!

Goodnight. I worship you and abominate this paper,
Always, your M.

1. On 12 September German airborne troops rescued Mussolini and flew him to Munich. Hitler ostensibly restored him to power and at Salo on Lake Garda he proclaimed the Fascist social republic.

Margaret to Tam — Two Gates, 15 September 1943

My Beloved,

All I can think of at the moment is the news. I can't help feeling that in spite of the Armistice[1] we are still in a pretty tight corner in Italy. What fools to let Musso slip through our fingers. He can still do a lot of harm, like one of our Australian snakes, even if you do cut it in two, the head is still dangerous for it can come back and join its other half. My silly old inside still playing up, don't suppose I could be having the change, could I? You'd better hurry back and help make Hedda[2] darling. Doctors say it is something left over from Hugo, but not at all serious and I feel quite well, so don't give it a thought. Seriously darling.

Hugo keeps us occupied, he really is a little boy now and sadly I say it, there is very little baby left, except late at night or when he really hurts himself.

Have sent off two small parcels darling, books, magazines, razor blades, soap, chocolate, benzedrine!!! So keep your eyes open for them my Tamèd. Hugo sleeps and Nanny and Mummy sew and I write to you and then go up and sleep with your old dressing gown. Always my love, ALWAYS, M.

1. King Victor Emanuel appointed Marshall Pietro Badoglio as Mussolini's successor and on 3 September the latter signed a secret armistice with the Allies.
2. The name they hoped to give their next baby.

Tam to Margaret Tarranto, Italy, 16 September 1943

My Darling,

If only these vile little foolscaps were not subject to censor and camera – still rather groggy from disappointment and contrite I mentioned anything about coming home.

Our meals are ludicrous. I have by fraternising madly, secured a case of champagne, a case of brandy, some gin and a bottle of Yellow Chartreuse, which helps down the everlasting Bully. Grapes, walnuts, figs in abundance. Very warm and fly blown and some really splendid smells. Take care of yourself, the more you write the more likely I shall get some of them. My love to Hugo and always to you my darling,
Tam

P.S. Bought you 18 pairs of silk stockings yesterday.

By the time Tam arrived in Italy the Allies had captured Salerno and Brindisi, giving them a line across the country from toe to heel, and were moving on Naples.

Tam to Margaret Tarranto, 23 September 1943

Oh my Beloved,

Why aren't you here in this musical comedy land of azure skies and seas. We should laugh so loud and long. Will try to give you an outline of what's been happening. Sailed from Bizerte in a beautiful cruiser on September 11th arriving Tarranto the following evening. After 72 hours of real Army balls up it was staggering to meet naval efficiency, but cruisers are hot little ships and we sweated incessantly. No Gin, but a bath. Slept on deck under a ground sheet with the spray from her bows drying on my face. A full moon which looked quite touchable.

Landing in the dark, a complete shambles. Lost half of my kit (FUCK) and were marched off in the wrong direction. Finally slept in an olive grove sans bed, sans blanket, sans mosquito net, sans everything. Bitten appallingly. Milk chocolate and Whisky for breakfast. Populace delighted at our arrival and we were soon showered with grapes the size of plums – wonderful. Moved again the next day which was spent in requisitioning vehicles. I got a Fiat which broke and now have a Lancia. The other day I arrived at an Italian General's H.Q., at least thirty men outside clicked their heels with an enormous amount of noise, flung their rifles from shoulder to shoulder, saluted and bowed. At the same moment the horn from my car started blowing and couldn't be stopped for twenty minutes. Stayed in lovely Hotel in Bari, was recognised! Grand Artista!! Eggs for breakfast, a manicure for twopence and tremendous service and attention, until I left a tap on and flooded a whole floor.

Made friends with a blue-eyed rascal in Tarranto (he's been in Hollywood, Manny Chevalier's[1] stand in). Offered me everything, his personal service, women and chicken lunch on Sunday at his villa in the country. Also suggested opening an Information Bureau for the Troops. Took him to the Military Police who thought it was an excellent plan. Next day he was arrested for changing B.M.A. (British Military Authority Currency) before the rate of exchange had been fixed. Fleecing the Troops badly. No chicken. Musical comedy gives way to Drama.

Just been ordered to move in two hours and have nothing to put eight men and all equipment and stores in except my little Lancia. This must be finished later, I have all the furniture to return to the Brothel. I love you so much, so much.

A little later

Now it's 'Alice in Wonderland' with a strong Marx Bros tendency. Just had a message marked 'Secret' everywhere, telling me if an Italian comes up and says 'Alba di Roma' and / or 'Orrani il Grane e mature' he's reliable, which is capital.

Later

I got all packed and then the order was cancelled. Luckily I hadn't returned the furniture. And so it goes on. Before long things will clarify but really since we landed things have been chaos. We were practically the first troops here and I've never before seen the beginning of a racket. The Lire is 400 to the £1 and I managed to get your stockings, a lot of drink and odds and ends before the prices went soaring. How long this campaign will last I've no idea, maybe till Christmas. Can't bear working for this Squadron after 'K'.[2] No organisation or control and they're a flappy crowd and not very cheerful when things are tiresome. I'm only with them for this job so will try like hell to come home as soon as it is over.

The Bosche have blown an aquaduct north of here and all sewers ceased to function at 8 this morning. Civilian latrines all along the sea front. Should be delightful in a couple of days.
All my love to Hugo and always and always to you, Tam

1. Maurice Chevalier (1881–1972), French actor and singer.
2. At the end of the North African campaign K squadron was disbanded and its members used to augment the numbers of H Squadron.

Margaret to Tam Two Gates, 29 September 1943

My Beloved,

Was quite unable to do a thing for a few days after your letter arrived saying it was definite you were not coming home my darling. Oh Golly, I don't think I ever really knew what the word disappointment meant till then. For days my mind and heart were in a whirl of joy, plans and excitement and then crash it all ended. I'm glad darling, as I said before, you got good and tight. I did too. Where are you my beloved, my treasure? It will be you for always and ever my love, so please be careful and come flying home to me as soon as you possibly can, we'll have such fun!

The news is still wonderful, both from Italy and Russia.[1] Golly, the Russians are only 60 miles from the Germans' own soil. Soon my love, soon I pray.
Keep the thought of our future and our love close to you,
All our love ALWAYS,
Hugo and M.

1. The Russian Army entered Kiev on 26 September and four days later the Allies took Naples, driving the enemy further north.

Tam to Margaret Italy, 30 September 1943

My darling,

So much of interest to tell you, and so little time and space. My last letter I think was written from Tarranto. Now much further north, beyond Foggia which has been featured the last two days by the B.B.C. We were there actually twenty four hours before they announced it. Utter desolation. Not a building left, nothing but glass, debris, and emaciated cats. I saw about ten civilians. This is a town the size of Windsor. One very old man raised his hat to me, which considering his entire town had been completely destroyed – so destroyed that if you rebuilt it you might just as well begin on some other site thirty miles away – I thought showed an irritating courtesy. In each village young children clap and cheer and people throw grapes into the jeep, and one is left with a purple stain down the front of one's shirt. Hundreds of refugees pouring south – terrible sights. Why do humans cling to worthless possessions? And all tramps in England have provided themselves with prams to carry their encumbrances about in. Not so here – everything in bundles, parcels, suitcases.

All this nonsense in the papers about Italy's war effort, iron wedding rings etc, must have been the most appalling cock. Quite obviously they never intended to try, and now they are delighted they haven't got to pretend to try any longer. Everything appeals to either one's sense of the dramatic or the ridiculous. One laughs at them and pities them.

Many escapists[1] coming through, very interesting. One said he'd ring you when he gets to England. Name McGibbon Lewis. Put in the bag in Crete. I bought him a room in the Hotel in Bari, dinner, champagne and a session at the barbers, so I dare say he will. Very nervy but overjoyed.

General opinion the enemy will attempt to hold a line south of Rome right across to Pescaro. My view they can't hold anything. They've no aircraft. I put the end of the war as any day after Christmas.

I rather think I was a sucker the other day in Bari. I got thirteen aquamarines, enough for a bracelet, nicely cut and matched, colour not very good. Cost 1850 liras, about £4. 12. 6d. If they don't fade or turn out to be glass they must surely be worth £50.

What is Noël Coward doing singing 'Don't let's be beastly to the Germans?' Will England ever be sane – it really shouldn't be tolerated. He should write a little ditty about the woman – eight months pregnant – who was slashed open, had the child ripped out and was left to die. This is a current and very popular story in Italy. I've heard it several times about Yugoslavia and Greece. Don't believe it. But I do believe all this shit which I can see and smell and is at my elbow, and which the Nazis didn't bury, and which I had to, and I shall be beastly to Germans always, and I hope so will my children, and if he continues to sing that song I shall be

beastly to Mr Coward. Maybe I'm being silly and it's great fun and very witty – here it annoys. Very well and fit,
Always and always,
Tam

1. Escaped prisoners-of-war.

Tam to Margaret Italy, 9 October 1943

Five weeks since I had a letter from you. Bloody not knowing what's happening or how you are. These confounded things take so long to reach you it's hopeless to give you news. Many rumours about. Continually on the move, which is something. The Aquamarines turned out to be phoney so I made the man take them back. Pity. They looked alright and as the price of a tart I understand is 7d, 7/6 for a small aquamarine seemed about right. Keep well and warm. Missing you a lot my darling. Cigarettes terribly short. Awful.
Always, Tam

Margaret to Tam Two Gates, 18 October 1943

My Tamèd,

Johnny has been here for the weekend, he seems very depressed and fed up with still hanging about. I think it's a mild attack of war nerves, poor old boy and a bit of the usual misery of going back after leave.

Hugo is wonderful and full of beans and talk. He has an old stick of yours which he will not be parted from, calls it 'Dada tick'. It is unfortunate too that he is mad about clocks and calls them cock. With the result that he shouts about cocks every time he sees a man because he has always seen them on men. If one makes him say please to see one the result is cock psss. Not good and I'm afraid it makes me laugh.

Golly golly golly darling what about the aquamarines, how exciting and wonderful and I must say they sound quite cheap. Thank you my love you are so sweet to think of buying me presents when you are in the midst of so much filth. I promise you that one day everything will be clean and delicious and pretty for you and I will too if I don't fade or lose my few looks. Oh how long, oh Lord how long. I do so hope the Hun does not make a long stand in Italy. The Volturno battle sounds very grim,[1] I wonder if casualties

are bad. Do take care of yourself darling. We are all well and fit and thinking of you all the time my dearest dearest. Love forever and always,
Your own M.

1. On 14 October the Allies broke through the German defence lines along the River Volturno.

Margaret to Tam Two Gates, 18 October 1943

My Beloved,

I keep on dashing these air letters off to you because I think they are the best by far. Went to London yesterday to get old Hugo some shoes and winter vests. Saw Rex and Lilli[1] in the Berkeley. Rex keeps his cap on all the time even in the bar – getting pretty thin on top methinks! Perhaps he'll wear uniform all the time after it's over. Lilli does not produce until next year. It seems ages since we all knew about it and she looks O.K. still. Golly I wish we were having our next darling. The amount I miss you seems to grow and grow, I do so long to see you darling.

Also went to see Ivan Smith, he is head of the Pacific B.B.C. and I'm to do a talk in a week or two to Australia on 1943 wartime clothes, export, materials etc and then do occasional talks at 2 or 3 weekly intervals which will fill a gap. The film I made is now called *The Lamp Still Burns* and is opening at the Odeon on the 21st. Perhaps if I get any sort of notice at all I'll get another film.

Still laughing at Italy's declaration of war,[2] what possible difference can it make, however badly the Germans are treating the Vatican. Golly I'd love to talk to you and hear what you know. And I'll love you always my darling,
Your M.

1. Rex Harrison and his wife Lilli Palmer.
2. On October Italy made a complete *volteface* by declaring war on Germany.

Tam to Margaret Italy, 21 October 1943

Well my darling,

It's alright this time. After ten days or so of waiting and wondering and frenzied efforts on the part of Hugh Fraser to frustrate the War Office, we really are – I say again – we really are coming home. Can't tell how long it will take, but I think we can safely bank on having your birthday together. Let the family know and tell Connie for somehow I must make you some money quickly for I imagine if there's still a job in Phantom we shall be employed again by March. What a Christmas we'll have and by the next one this fucking war will be over.

Look lovely for me when I see you first. Five or six weeks I reckon, maybe via North Africa. Oh Darling, what bliss it will be. Take care of yourself till I can. Be good and don't get the 'phone cut off. My love for always and always,
Tam

On 21 October Tam's jeep went over a mine and his driver was killed. He had a lucky escape, suffering only from bruising and shock. It seems likely that he did not tell Margaret in order not to worry her, as the incident is not referred to in any of their letters..

Margaret to Tam — Two Gates, 25 October 1943

My angel, my beloved,

Today is Monday, I've not had a letter from you since the week before last. I do hope you are alright darling. I know that your letters from there *have* begun to arrive and unless you are moving about a lot and terribly busy – which I bet you are now, they should be coming in fairly regularly.

Noël Coward gave the post script to the news last night. He spoke about his recent tour of the Middle and Near East – the hospitals, camps etc he'd visited. Said he's been the guest of the Army, the Navy and the Air Force, had travelled far and wide and seen and learnt many things, all really a lot of cow towing in that clipped, should never leave London voice of his, and then came the real reason for the broadcast. He said a lot of people have taken exception to a recent song of mine 'Don't Let's Be Beastly to the Germans'. He went on to explain that he had meant it as a vitriolic satyr [*sic*] and that the people who had not understood it had perhaps an inadequate knowledge of the English language. Well all I can say is the title is unfortunate whatever the content.

Hugo is wonderful; his new saying is 'a bas mama' which means God Bless. I think it is rather a sweet way of saying it, don't you? He is as fit as a fiddle and still talks about Dada a lot. Take care of yourself my love, keep warm, here I'm waiting.
Always, Your M.

Margaret to Tam Two Gates, 26 October 1943

Beloved,

I've just read the papers and it says troops on the Continent are to have ten days' leave before Christmas, always providing there is not a big battle on. It also says length of service and previous service abroad men will have priority. Quite excited but I must keep a grip as it may not apply to you. Hugo is with me at the moment and as he never draws breath these days it is difficult to write darling. No Joyce to help and Mummy still in bed poor darling.

Hugo just heard me telephoning to Daniel Neal's for some red shoes for him and he shouted *no no no* Mummy I want black shoes to be like Daddy. He seems to think you wear a lot of black, maybe it is the hair. He never stops saying he wants black hair like you. More tonight my love, I adore you. Now for the lunch.
Always and always,
Your M.

Margaret to Tam Two Gates, 1 November 1943

AT LAST my Beloved, *at last.* Oh my darling what wonderful, glorious, happy, perfect news. I can say no more. I think I've told you many times in my letters how terribly much I miss you. It really is too perfect, and now that I know that, the waiting will seem unendurable. Just for safety I'd told myself – you may not see him for over a year, maybe more, so *wait*! And now the waiting's all over except for these next weeks of preparing. I told Hugo you were coming home and he looked at me hard for a moment, then said – Boat? Dada? I've always told him that you'd gone in a boat and now he asks if you are coming home the same way.

Bad luck darling about the aquamarines but really I don't care a fuck if you are coming home. I'm busying up to London tomorrow to try to extricate a few more pence from the bank. Quite a game! However, don't worry darling and don't imagine you are coming home to a load of debt, you are *not*, and it could be a lot worse. *I'm not worried*. Take great care of yourself. Wonder how you are coming and *really* how long you'll be.
I do love you so much,
For always,
Your M.

Tam to Margaret — Italy, 10 November 1943

My Darling,

Still sitting stupidly on our bottoms listening to the B.B.C. news and waiting impatiently. But it won't be long now, and any time now after December 1st you must leave your telephone number if you go to London. Heard Churchill last night promising a blood bath next year.[1] But I fancy the most important news of the week is that Stalin says the liberated must have self chosen government.[2] I've been thinking a great deal about after the war lately – it seems inevitable that we shall be miserably poor, my pretty – anyway until the girls are grown up – then maybe we'll have a couple of years respite until ours start. But I see an endless vista of exhausting expenses – but I don't care as long as you don't.

Darling I am concerned at the disappointment you will feel at my appearance. After nearly a year of looking at Dorothy Wilding's flattering picture of 1939 I fear you will be horrified at the wizened, white-haired, toothless, rather yellow little monster I have become. Is our son showing any signs of good looks or is he still half Beaverbrook, half monoplane? How I look forward to seeing him. Prue is leaving Cheltenham Ladies' College and is to have a long course of osteopathy, but they say she can return later.[3] God bless you my darling, see you soon,

Always and always,

Tam

1. The nation was becoming impatient about the long-anticipated invasion of France. Churchill was doubtless pandering to this.
2. An important gesture, not fulfilled. The Allies were concerned that Russia would bring all the lands she had liberated under Communist rule.
3. Prue had severe asthma and it was thought a course of osteopathy might bring her relief.

Margaret to Tam — Two Gates, 10 December 1943

My love, my Tam,

Having been entirely eaten up with excitement and anticipation and joy of looking forward to seeing you before Xmas, today I suffered the bitterest disappointment of my life. 12 fucking P. boys home and not a sign of you.[1] Golly I thought my heart would break and then I thought of you my darling and how disappointed you too must be. I just can't think about it. And now I've missed the chance of sending you anything for Christmas, even this sad,

defeated and disappointed little letter may not reach you in time after it has buggered all over the country looking for you. I'm told you will not be here early in the N. Year. Jan 8th perhaps? Remember my beloved? Where oh where will you be my love? Somewhere where you can get a good meal and plenty of alcohol.
Always, Your M.

1. Tam was not amongst the Phantom Officers home on leave.

Tam to Margaret Algiers, 13 December 1943

My darling,

This I hope is the last time I shall have to write my Happy Christmas to you. Every known kind of delay and disappointment and hinderance and annoyance has attended us and I'm filled with a sulky despair, and general loathing for all human kind. I suppose I am like my darling mother who is at her worst when frustrated. After the most ghastly train journey of four and a half days we arrived at a Transit Camp in a little resort called Blida – the i is pronounced so rightly as double e – however we've escaped from there and are now on a farm and independent. Needless to say I hadn't been here for twenty-four hours before I fixed myself a 'plane home – but Hugh Fraser, in spite of my entreaties, wouldn't let me go. So here we sit waiting for our ship to come in – some say early in the New Year, and I heard yesterday wild rumours of a three week quarantine on arrival. It is now over two months since we started to leave. Added to all the other horrors Christmas Theatricals have cropped up, which really have crowned my ultimate unhappiness. I've tried to cable you, and I've tried getting away and now there's nothing left to do but endure the boredom. I have luckily made friends with a little fellow who can keep me supplied with with a sufficiency of Algerian brandy, and I anticipate the major part of my waking hours will be spent in pain and hangover. I've never wanted you so badly, and never missed you so much. I'm bored and unhappy and disappointed, frustrated and wretched. But next year my love this will seem unimportant and very distant and we shall laugh at it above the tinkle of the ice. Perhaps if I tell you, that after an hour and a half of forceful arguments I have just succeeded in squashing an idea to produce an abbreviated version of *A Midsummer Night's Dream* – to be produced by the end of the week without wigs, costumes, stage, or lighting, and only one copy of the play, you may appreciate the

nervous exhaustion I suffer. Don't worry I'm well and expect me when you see me. I'll be much nicer in my next letter,
Always and always,
Tam

Tam to Margaret Algiers, 16 December 1943

Darling,

Two letters from you an hour or so ago telling me you knew the maddening news, which is a relief for I've been worrying that you'd be worried. I rather think my last letter to you a few days ago will not reach you, for some silly bugger posted it without a stamp. So a Happy Christmas once more my darling Margaret – next year there'll be no blackout, no separation and Hugo will come into our bed in the morning pink and hot with excitement and we shall make the supreme parental effort and become excited too.

Cold here now – I'm back to dressing up to go to bed again. I consider it long odds in misfortune to spend two Christmases in Algiers. Thirty two years ago Mum and I were here.

God in his great wisdom and infinite mercy has given me an idea to frustrate the Officers performing *Cinderella*. I have toiled to wig makers and costumiers and estimated the cost of production at over £20. But I liked my title – *More sinned against than Cinderella* – and whisper who dares – tonight, maybe tomorrow, in borrowed civilian clothes I may be turning up a nine or two, for we've discovered the Casino. The nines will have to present themselves fairly promptly, otherwise my visit will be a matter of minutes. I think of nothing but seeing you – amongst other things in my suit – and of all the happiness so nearly there. I love you so much. Be good sweet maid and let who will be sober – wait impatiently for me – and what's your telephone number please?
Always and always,
Tam

1944–5

Margaret to Tam Two Gates, 8 January 1944

My Darling,

Seven years ago today, Gotham, New York. What a lovely night that was, what fun we had my darling. Shall we do it all over again?

The little verse you wrote for me arrived this morning. Thank you my darling I love it and I'm very proud that you should write such sweetness to me still. Please love me always. I did write you a letter for our day and if my letters are reaching you as fast as yours are coming now, you should have received it. I hope so. I have not written you a verse because I found the Marquis of Crewe had kindly done it for me.

You were most interesting about *Henry V*[1] and so was your Mum who said he lacked humour and fire. The humour particularly in the love scenes. But no doubt she has written to you about it. I have not seen it yet but hope to go this week.

I need hardly tell you that the optimism re the war cheers me a lot because I am at the moment very low and depressed. I have a feeling things are going rather badly and of course they've succeeded in bitching our plans for the future if nothing else. Thank you for the verse again darling. I love it and I love you too more than I'll ever be able to tell you.

Always and Always,
Your M.

1. Laurence Olivier's film of *Henry V*. Later Olivier credited Tam with giving him the idea for the film.

Seven Years
By the Marquess of Crewe

To join the ages they have gone,
Those seven years,
Receding as the months roll on,
Yet very oft my fancy hears
Your voice – 'Twas music to my ears
Those seven years.

Scant the shadow and high the sun,
Those seven years,
Can hearts be one, then ours were one,
One for laughter and one for tears
Knit together in hopes and fears,
Those seven years.

How, perchance, do they seem to you,
  Those seven years,
Spirit free in the wider blue?
When time and eternity disappears
What if all you have learn'd but the more endears
  Those seven years.

And this with all my love beloved.

After a period of leave Tam spent the early part of 1944 stationed at Matlock in Derbyshire, while the Allies prepared for the D-Day landings in Normandy. Though still serving in Phantom, he was put under contract to the film producer Alexander Korda but, to his continuing frustration, was not released to make a picture.

Margaret to Tam Two Gates, Shrove Tuesday 1944

My own beloved,

We have just had pancakes and I'm now warm for the first time today. Golly that studio is cold, but never mind it was another day and that makes four.[1] As you know, two days in a studio gives one no news, so I have none.

Oh my love I do miss you. Hope you did not have too bad a journey and were not too cold. Are you fairly comfortable, I wonder, and is there anyone amusing for you to talk to?

Good news from Russia tonight,[2] but I don't understand why Hitler has decided to defend Rome so strongly.[3] They said on the news he'd sent eighteen more divisions there – and the weather there is lousy again. And now old Churchill is warning us against optimism again – so what! I wonder will it end this year, I wonder? Oh my love, it must. I shall have your Prue next week end and the next one you will be home, oh happy day.

Take care of yourself my love, keep warm, love me and don't fret or worry too much please! We will be alright for you surely are a King who is loved adored and worshipped by a Princess in her own right. And I love you too.

Always and always, your M.

1. Margaret was filming *Give Me the Stars*.
2. After two weeks' fighting the Russians destroyed ten divisions of the German 8th Army trapped south-east of Kiev. 52,000 Germans were killed and 11,000 taken prisoner.
3. For four months the Germans defended Monte Cassino which was blocking the Allies' route to Rome. There was also fierce fighting when the Allies landed troops on the beach at Anzio, north of Cassino.

Margaret to Tam — Two Gates, 15 March 1944

Well my most beloved, how are you and where I wonder are you? Mummy and Joyce have gone to see Greer Garson and Walter Pidgeon in *Mrs Parkington*. I think I told you I saw it earlier in the week with Vi and Charles. It stinks, oh golly it is so slow. Mr Pidgeon is dull dull dull. However in spite of this and more which I told them, off they've gone so I've got myself to myself. The most lovely sunny day here today. Bought some seeds for the garden and Joyce and I are going to get to work in earnest. Lettuce, carrots, onions, radishes etc. Hugo helps (?) with his small wheelbarrow and looks very important about it.

Oh gosh, I'd quite forgotten to tell you about my party last night. Vi and Charles went to London; drove us all the way up and back in a Lancia. We dined at Bates which is now a dinner and dance place since poker and bridge are illegal. Then we went to the Milroy (the place you call an aquarium) where we stayed until about one o'clock. Saw Jack Profumo, it was grand to see him, he was so gay and jolly and glad to be in London and was *of course* with the prettiest girl in town, Pam Rank, the only snag about her being that she won't budge out of her door for any but the very rich! I had a dance with him and he sent you his very best. He is off back to Italy in a day or two. Says he'll be back in three months. Home and in bed by just after two.

Darling write me a nice long loving letter as soon as you have enough time. Take care of yourself and always remember I love you love you love you. Your own Maggy.

Tam was allowed home for a few days' leave prior to going overseas again, this time to Normandy, as part of the Allied invasion of France which commenced on 6 June.

Margaret to Tam — London, 4 May 1944

Oh my darling sweetheart,

What a truly happy and lovely time we had together yesterday. I *did* so enjoy myself my love. You were wonderful and it was such heaven to be really truly alone for once. Let us do the same next time?

I haven't much news. A rude maid came thumping in at eight this morning and when I told her to get out and let me sleep she shouted and nattered about checking her rooms and having me out by ten and ended up by calling me tripe! Which I rather felt like I must say. However I reported her and went to sleep again. Had a call from the studio, so I'm working again tomorrow. Called at nine, so I'm off on the 6.40 train which is torture for me.

Oh my darling, how have you felt today? I'll bet you were tired after your night and then the train trip. You poor sweet. I thought of you all day and hoped you'd get a chance for a sleep. I absolutely adore you, you were wonderful last night,
Always and always,
Your M.

Tam to Margaret England, 8 May 1944

My Beloved,

I know this next time won't be so long and the whole future is considerably brighter than it was last year – but oh dear, I'm filled with such a melancholy when I think of being away from you again. Never again after the war, not even long weekends. I went to church and sat in the sun and for once lost this eve of the Derby feeling everyone is pumping into one. The people of the world may be fighting and warlike, but the earth itself has never seemed so peaceful and fruitful and perfect as this April. I found this in *The Vicar of Wakefield* yesterday. I quote it to you not as the sum total of my post-war desires for though forty I'm not yet a fogey – but as most of what I want. It's English and home and happiness and peace of mind, which by God's miracle it looks as if we shall achieve. I really did give thanks in church this morning – here it is.

'We had an elegant house in a good neighbourhood, we had no revolutions to fear, nor fatigues to undergo; all our adventures were by the fire side, and all our migrations from the blue bed to the brown.'

Isn't it charming and so utterly enviable, and again:

'We kept up the Christmas Carol, sent true love knots on Valentine morning, ate pancakes on Shrovetide, shewed our wit on the 1st of April and religiously cracked nuts on Michaelmas Eve.' There's the English cycle complete. That's how Hugo must find the world.
Always and always my darling,
Tam

Margaret to Tam — Two Gates, 17 June 1944

My Beloved,

I wonder just whereabouts in France you are and how you are getting on. I gather you are now moved from the white cliffs and dealing in francs, that you are doing a good job very well and that the Col. is very pleased with you. Wonder did you have a tricky crossing, and what sort of landing you made and where? Oh dear, I seem to wonder about you all day long my darling. Which is to say I miss you more than ever before.

What about these new rocket bomb planes,[1] rather frightening I think, on account of they may go *anywhere*. How can they completely control such things. I hear a pub in old Windsor was hit the other night. Quite flat. The news from France is better today, the Cherbourg peninsula is cut off all but ten miles and all the winter offensives are well held.[2] Weather bad for the air though, which is bad of course. Oh darling surely it won't be long this time before we can be together again. Christmas for sure I'd say.

Nanny and Mummy say to send you their best love,

And forever and always darling from Hugo and me, your M.

1. On 14 June the first V1 flying bombs reached England. Given the nickname of 'Doodlebug' or 'Buzzbomb', they were pilot-less, jet-propelled, and could deliver nearly a ton of high explosive.
2. The Allies launched a massive invasion of Normandy on 6 June. By the 12th the five main beach heads had been linked to form a continuous front. General Montgomery and the British sought to draw the Germans into the Caen sector and take some pressure off the Americans in the well-defended Cherbourg Peninsula. By 27 June the town of Cherbourg was taken.

Tam to Margaret — On arrival in Normandy, 17 June 1944

I arrived late last night after a comfortable but lengthy crossing. Personally I prefer the Riviera, but this isn't bad – very crowded of course, but the weather is perfect. In Africa and Italy you and everything else in England seemed so very far and distant, but here it's different and I have the quite ridiculous feeling that I might dine in London – it'll wear off no doubt. My position here is tricky in the extreme – enormous tact necessary to get anything – which slows everything up damnably. However it will improve. At the moment I have no transport, no tent, not a map, not a pencil of my own, for my patrol doesn't arrive until next week sometime. I want so much to make a success of it for it was my idea I came ahead. At last my love I am a Captain! What rank that makes me at Aspreys where I've been a Major since 1941 I can't quite work out.

This may with luck reach you on the 21st. If so my darling as many times as possible I shall be thinking of you and wishing I were with you. Next Year. Pray God this is the last year I shall keep writing 'next year'. A little noisy here last night, particularly a nervous cow that is tethered near my hole in the ground. Write often my best beloved,
Always and always,
Tam

I failed to get this off yesterday so will add a line or two. I had a strange landing. So many times arriving or leaving places it would have been comforting to have been recognised, but as a rule the Press – if any – click their little bored cameras for pictures which are never published, and the handful of people idly watching wonder who the hell one is. But staggering up the beach with my valise and packs, overcoat, tin hat and gas mask I asked a soldier if he would give me a hand – 'Certainly Mr Williams if I can have your autograph' – I must have signed about thirty and have never felt such an old ham in my life. I'd been rather working myself up too – Henry V and all sorts – I'm always de-bunked so flat when I begin to dramatise.

I have an A.A. Battery under my pillow otherwise fairly comfortable,
My love forever and always,
Tam

(Have you heard this description of the beach on D-Day, 'My dear *everyone* was there!' Don't stay in London until they've got those pilotless things taped, or is it really not as bad as it sounds?).

Tam to Margaret — Normandy, 22 June 1944

My Darling,

Did I give you this new address yesterday? B.W.E.F. No one knows what the letters stand for. The best I can do with it is Buggered With Effect From.

I find it difficult to write – there is only one subject and that's impossible. I found this in my W.E.Henley[1], which I wish could have reached you yesterday. Did you get some flowers from me?

'Across the miles between us
I send you sigh for sigh.
Good night, sweet friend, good night;
'Til life and all take flight,
Never goodbye.'

How's my Hugo? How like heaven that miserable little cottage seems. Noisy here and very crowded. God bless you I love you my pretty – take care great care – seems a lot more than two weeks since I saw you,
Always and always,
Tam

1. From the sequence of poems 'Hawthorn and Lavender' by W.E. Henley, published in 1901.

Tam to Margaret Normandy, 28 June 1944

My beloved,
Working rather strenuously as I said. With another Officer it would be splendid, as it is there's little time for anything but food and sleep – very dirty, only because I cannot and will not wash my armpits in a rainstorm. Be patient, we're nearly there. Christmas will see me a slick little civilian.

Went out with Johnny for a couple of hours yesterday – quite bad mud – midsummer wind like March, thunder storms like Ascot, rain like Wimbledon. Lots of dead cattle. Food very monotonous, but I think it's wonderful we have any. Americans I hear are being very generous about us – realising the greater difficulties on our Front, and giving us the credit for Cherbourg[1] – quite right. I hear plenty of Martell Three Star captured there – Phantom is ordering collection rapidly. Find I dream all night of messages – eighteen hours a day and I can't suddenly switch my mind off – then in the morning I'm confused as to what I've dreamt and what really happened. Sent some cheese off to you – should be très fort on arrival.
All my love always and always and to my Hugo,
Tam

1. The British successfully drew German troops away from Cherbourg by attacking Caen.

Tam to Margaret Normandy, 30 June 1944

My Darling,

Been having a very busy period – it's a damn tricky difficult job, and bloody hard work – the days come and last a long time and go without one's noticing. Had certain play with a goose yesterday, which wandered into our lines. It narrowly escaped death but we heard it belonged to the Army Commander and had been given to him by some Commandos who had made friends with it on D-Day, so finally we had to send it back. He had become very attached to it and regarded its disappearance as a bad omen. Aide de Camps and men sent in search and his whole camp was in an uproar, then one highly intelligent Sergeant merely seized the first large goose he saw and returned in triumph (with a French woman screaming in the distance) expecting a reward. Maddening – for the General would never have known the difference between two white geese and we could have had it tonight instead of a very liquid, very lukewarm greasy stew. If you ever get the parcel of cheese I sent, send the stamps on to Prudie will you? Wish I could send you some butter. Now the Bosche have stopped sending it all to Germany there's bags of it. Have worked out on a basis of pre-war prices that if you and I had half a bottle of the dear stuff each morning and a bottle at night, it would only cost us about 18/- a day.

God bless you my darling, my love always,

Tam

Margaret to Tam Two Gates, 2 July 1944

My Darling,

I've had rather a gay weekend for me. It is strange how a little fun makes one miss the great fun one had had. On Sunday after lunch we all went over to Clivedon [*sic*] to see Barbara Astor and Michael[1], who has been home since last Tuesday. They are taking it very easy I gather. Barbara asked me to go to Scotland with her. She is going next Tuesday for three weeks to an island called Duro they have. Plenty of eggs, butter, cream etc, and no radios, no papers, no telephone. It does sound the perfect rest I must say, but I just can't go and leave Hugo here. Clivedon is a heavenly place. I would love to spend a weekend there with you my love. We must get Barbara to ask us after the war.

Had a long talk to Gwynne on the telephone this morning. Prue is coming over here and I'm looking forward to seeing her very much. Poor child. G says she has had a touch of asthma all week, just when she was to have been in all the school events. Prue is always so very brave when her old asthma spoils her fun, I admire her so much. She says she is getting resigned now. I shall take her to the cinema or local theatre if suitable, or perhaps we'll bike over to Monkey Island.

The news this morning is terrific, the weekend seems to have brought successes on all three fronts.[2] I can't believe the Russians are beyond Minsk now.[3] I feel the fighting must be very hard and bitter round Caen though.[4] Oh darling how I wish could talk to you. But perhaps I won't have to wait so long this time, I pray not. Still the new toy of Hitler's keeps roaring over. It is a horrible thing and no one likes them, but I feel that they will be fixed before very long.

Take care my love and remember I'm thinking of you and I adore you.

Always and always,
Your M.

1. Captain the Honourable Michael Langhorne Astor (1916–80) served in Phantom with Tam. He married Barbara Colonsay who died in 1980.
2. On 4 June 1944 the Allies liberated Rome.
3. Minsk was the last big German base on Russian soil. The Russians had now breached the Germans' 'Fatherland Line' of defence in White Russia.
4. Montgomery was now meeting bloody resistance from the Germans around Caen.

Margaret to Tam — Two Gates, 5 July 1944

Darling One,

Still not going to London so yet another day of heavy domesticity. Went to the movies with Mummy and Eliza. Saw Tyrone Power in *The Mark of Zorro*, lots of black cloaks, masks and swordplay. Back again in time to say goodnight to our son. Jeremy Clyde[1] rang him up this morning – I went to the nursery and said a friend wanted to talk to him on the telephone – he *rushed* into my room, picked up the receiver and said 'Daddy?' My heart broke and his face *fell* when I said 'No darling, it's Jeremy and he wants you to go to tea.' So later I took him in my arms and explained that you would ring him one day soon, but not just yet. And he smiled and nodded and said 'Soon Mummy' and I said yes. He seems so keen on his Daddy these last few weeks. He is such a comfort darling, I do adore him and my only wish is to start another as soon as we can.

Your fourth letter arrived this morning, dated June 28th – saying you were dreaming messages. I know exactly what you mean, ghastly confusing. You poor sweet, I do admire your grit, and I promise you you shall be clean, rested (except for occasional hang-overs) and slick after the war my beloved. By Christmas? I wonder, I pray, I hope. Golly how well the map looks now, wonderful advances from Russia, Italy and France. Oh love, take care of yourself and get some rest soon, and remember I love and adore you,
Always and always, your own Margot.

1. Jeremy Clyde, small son of Eliza and Tommy Clyde, now an actor and still great friends with Hugo.

Tam to Margaret Normandy, 6 July 1944

My Darling,

Three letters from you today. Good news, Maurice MacMillan[1] is joining me so thank God I shall get some spells off – it's three weeks practically since I was not on duty and I've only been out of this field twice. Have been working till I'm practically red hot. The sun came out yesterday and I got in a bath. Have you been in touch with Chivers,[2] am I bankrupt or are they behaving decently?

I've seen Niven, he came in yesterday. Very amusing, very funny and fearfully embarrassing. The gags and the dialogue lasted just long enough and he was off. You'll hear it all I dare say, but when he gets to the one about asking the way somewhere down near the front, having map-read rather badly, and getting the answer in German from a head poked out of a tank, just say, 'Yes that really did happen, but to an ambulance driver in Hottot.' He got away with it by the way and got back.

I hear they double censor letters now which is causing fearful delays – I've written at least three times a week. Have you got any parcels yet, and in what condition did they arrive?
Always and always, Tam

1. Captain Maurice Macmillan, son of future Prime Minister Harold Macmillan and later an MP himself.
2. Tam and Margaret's accountant who was handling on-going difficulties with the Inland Revenue about income tax that Tam owed.

Margaret to Tam — Two Gates, 7 July 1944

Tamèd my darling,

It is just 11.15 and Nanny has just got in from seeing *Gone With The Wind* again. A real endurance test. Mummy and I have been sitting reading and listening to the heavy continuous roar of our airplanes over head. The numbers of planes seem to grow each day. Lucky planes for some of them will be nearer to you than me tonight. Some evenings as I write to you the yearning in me for a sight of you becomes so intense that I can almost feel you beside me. I suppose really we are not far apart at moments like this darling.

Sirens have been going on and off all evening, but so far we've only heard one bump, some way off I hope!! Did you read Churchill's speech on the new so-called missiles, not very reassuring but what can the poor man say? No one likes them and they are beastly, let's face it. Hope your part of the world is not getting them darling.

Chivers rang to say that the Income Tax wished to see you and were still fairly determined. However I said you were in France and Chivers seemed to think this might be in our favour for the time being. He said he would keep in touch with me and would appreciate a cheque for himself as soon as possible. I'm getting writer's cramp from staving off creditors.

Had dinner last night with a large rather common man Capt Anthony Hume. Met him at Vi's party. Really quite nice and kind and he certainly gave me a nice dinner (at the Brook Club, Ascot). I'm afraid I talked about you all night darling, so I don't suppose I'll be asked again. I seem to remember that men are not mad about having another man shoved down their throats all evening. Anyhow I brought him home at 11.30 and gave him a cup of tea in the bosom of my family.

Still have some lovely cheese left, it is delicious darling and thank you again. Have sent 200 cigs a week to you my love, they are called Sunripe. I've only ordered a month so let me know if you like them.

This letter will be a bore if I go on much longer my love, so I send you all our love, Hugo's and mine,
For always and always,
Your own M.

Tam to Margaret Normandy, 7 July 1944

My Darling,

If my letters are dull forgive me, when I put pen to paper now my instinct is to write some terrible military gibberish. I managed to dart into the town this afternoon and get a couple of lengths of some not very rich but quite gay material, and some rather nice stuff for shirts for you. Not a bottle of Cognac or wine in the place – I tried six wholesale places – their ration is one litre per month. The Bosche never dealt with the small people, they requisitioned what they wanted from the top – 10,000 cases of Martell per week. One of my clauses in the Peace terms is that no German shall drink French wine for a hundred years and all their hocks shall be exported free to the Allies. Everyone I talked to was charming but rather gave one the feeling one was a fool to ask for wine and that surely one knew the Bosche had had it all. They tell me it will be the same as we get further south which depressed me dreadfully. It's bad to have gone through two lousy wine growing countries like North Africa and Italy and at last to reach France and find the cupboard bare. Does Hugo really talk about me? Bless his darling heart, keep him going. If David Niven comes back again make him bring me a bottle.

I'll have a bit more time after tomorrow when Maurice arrives. God bless you always and always,

Tam

Margaret to Tam Two Gates, 9 July 1944

My Love,

Did not write yesterday because I was a bit tiddly when I came home. First of all Charles[1] arrived back from London with your parcel. Darling you are a thoughtful, remembering husband, everything was lovely and all the things I wanted bless you. Thank you. The combs I was in desperate need of, the scent is lovely but try for Patou next time!! Talc and face powder perfect. Poor old Niven got some *filth* for Prim. Last night he rang and said he'd seen you and would I go round for a drink to hear the news, so I did. It was grand to hear about you my love and to know you were well. He said you were on magnificent form, but I couldn't help wondering if it had been an act you were putting on. It sounded as if you were bloody uncomfortable and *no* drink. I'm seeing to that *at once*. David said he'd taken photographs of you and Johnny, longing to see them. He nattered away about all he'd seen but I felt he only saw the gravy or the top of the milk, and I felt from his talk that you'd been gay but not opened up to him much. Was I right? And just what was he up to? Prim put on such an act when he left and fled to Leicester from the bombs – what bombs? – *really*! All that stuff about being alone in the house if and when the fated news came. I should think if such news ever did come the only possible thing would to be to be alone. However with all my chat I was happy to get direct news of you my precious. I'm so in love with you. Curse arrived yesterday, so that is that. Oh darling I can't ever tell you how I *long* to start another baby. Next time we must try even harder. I only regret that Hugo will be so much older than Hedda, but I suppose it won't matter. I'm off to Dr Maxwell as soon as I'm O.K., I'm sure there is nothing really wrong, because I don't feel ill or anything as I would if there were. Maybe God thought we should wait a bit, because he sent us Hugo at a moment when only He could have known it was right, didn't he? So maybe our next baby will be the same darling. Anyhow we'll be together all our lives when this bloody war is over, so we've a lot of time haven't we my love?

I'm fond and loving and waiting beloved, so don't ever worry about me, and let me know the moment you want anything. Hugo said this morning, 'One day Daddy will put down his gun and pick up his umdum' (umbrella) I was flabbergasted. What do you make of that? We both adore you and I personally will love you for always and always,

Your own M.

1. Lieutenant Lord Charles Banbury, known as 'The Bag', serving in Phantom and a friend of Tam's.

Margaret to Tam — Two Gates, 11 July 1944

Beloved,

Thank you my love for going shopping and buying me a present, I can't wait to see what you got, but Tam darling don't spend your precious money buying me presents, get yourself something you want or save it for a bit of a 'Do' in Paris. I'll look up some addresses for you, some may still be the same. I mean, of course, a dancing and drinking party, the other is reserved for us.

It's strange how the time goes marching by and one day merges into a week, and a week into a month without somehow being much noticed. I suppose it is having so little to look forward to other than the end of the war and having you home again. One's entire physical and emotional being becomes focused on one spot and remains there. What happens in between seems to be just part of a rather mixed up dream. You and what you mean are reality. This is all nonsense except for Hugo and his charm and his happiness and concern for his welfare. To write to you these days is my joy, my escape and I just cosy down with my pen and try to talk to you. It's a pity that my prose is not better and that I am not more eloquent, else my letters would be worth keeping.

I still think we've a long way to go and the map looks colossal to me in spite of the glorious advances and successes on all fronts. Caen news of course has been truly thrilling[1] and I'll bet you had an oddly fascinating 3 or 4 days. More tomorrow my love, to bed now. God bless and keep you safe, always and always, your M.

1. On 9 July Caen fell to the Allies.

Tam to Margaret — Normandy, 14 July 1944

Darling,

An altogether charming memory this morning. Quatorze Juillet the Mayor of the nearby village and some small children presented Johnny with a bunch of flowers tied up with the Tricolour. Vive la France and three cheers, a glass of wine and chocolate for the kids – I thought it would be frightfully funny – but found it very touching. A little boy almost Hugo's size had been slightly wounded by shrapnel and all the rest had lost either mother or father. I have been thinking awfully seriously the last two or three days about you're going further away from the doodle bombs. Take a cottage in Wales or Cornwall or the Cotswolds and write off the next three months as an absolute waste of time – be patient and wait. When there is no possible reason to stay in the danger area I cannot see that it is anything but stupid to do so – go to the sea somewhere, take some books and some tapestry work and drive yourself crazy. It's like throwing darts – if you have enough turns sooner or later the whole board has a mark on it. Think it over most carefully. I believe they've got more of the bloody things up their sleeve. I shall be back by November and we can start life again. Well not really again, for we've never had a go yet have we?

All my love for you and always and to the boy,

Tam

Margaret to Tam — Two Gates, 18 July 1944

Oh darling,

Wonderful news of another big attack tonight. I can gather that once Caen is taken there will be quite a big advance towards Paris. The Russians careering towards E. Prussia, you towards Paris and the 5th and 8th storming northwards. That sounds as if you and you alone are coping with Normandy. Well I suppose in my heart of hearts you are my one thought when I hear the news darling, and thus I suppose it is in every woman's heart about at least one man, so in such a way the units are made the mass and so all are taken care of in the prayers we say.

Hugo wrote to you and put the letter in the post today himself. But I doubt you will get it as it was only a scribble on a piece of odd paper I'd given him.

Do you really think you'll be with us by Nov. darling one? If only I could believe that. Yes darling, we will start to live and make plans. I think we'll be broke sometimes but let us hope it will be a full life and a gay yet cosy one. How I'd love to sit and drink with you tonight.

It is now 10.30 and I'm going to have an early night and good sleep. God bless and keep you. Oh did I tell you that I've sent two bottles over for you? I think David is a bad bet, don't believe he'll go again if he can help it, and Prim does not like it!!

Goodnight my love and remember I adore you for always,

Your M.

Tam to Margaret — Normandy, 22 July 1944

Darling,

Haven't written for a couple of days, mainly because it's not ceased raining – everything leaking and muddy and damp and dripping and limp. Yesterday was so peculiarly unattractive that Johnny and I set about our month's supply of whisky and reduced it to nothing before retiring between wet and dirty sheets. Very pleasant, and it made me quite nostalgic having a hangover once more. Someone should start a school in post war England for training assasins [*sic*][1] – they invariably miss. Mussolini years ago. Laval and now Hitler. I hear Rex Whistler[2] has been killed – a great pity and a great loss.

Take care. Be good and love me a great deal. All my love to you always and always,
Tam

1. On 20 July three German officers were killed during an attempt on the Führer's life. Colonel Graf Klaus was accused of planting a suitcase bomb in Hitler's Conference Room, and was hanged.
2. Rex John Whistler (1905–44), English artist and set designer.

Tam to Margaret Normandy, 31 July 1944

My darling,
A real summer day with the blessed blue sky all the way round and the third eleven scoring very freely again this morning after a good start yesterday. My servant has contact with a farm woman for one egg a day for me and my laundry each week, so I had it boiled for my breakfast and clean sheets tonight – so it's long odds on we shall move shortly with such a coup as that in my pocket. I've been offered – by a greedier and less thirsty officer – two large whiskies for my egg this evening – a deal I closed on the instant being very much in need, for yesterday was very long and today promises the same way. I shall take them both together with very little water as I get to my bed – then I'll sleep beautifully – otherwise I'm very apt to write and telephone messages until I sharpen my pencil again in the morning. Tell Hugo my patrol has a rabbit – MINNIE – a fat old girl in black and white – and she sits in the sun and fools around all day and is very difficult to catch in the evening to put in her house. Candles would be very useful, also Enos, sorry to keep asking you for things but one is so dependent on you and you're so sweet and pretty and clever I know you don't mind – you be good too. I shall love you always and always,
My adorable Margaret, your ever loving Celandine.

Tam to Margaret Normandy, 3 August 1944

My darling,
A very busy week as you've probably guessed. Good news all the time – but have had little time to write to you. Very comfortable in my tent now – reading light and large mirror. And my egg supply is now two a day. Minnie is nearing her time and getting very fat. Very optimistic about everything – ugly rumours about Phantom

going to Burma – not me my darling – Sir Alexander[1] will claim me I trust. But I reckon twelve weeks will see it finished. Missing you terribly, physically much more than last time. Are you behaving? Not long to wait my pretty. The bloody French. No more wine, cheese or butter and we're not allowed in any restaurants from now till further notice. Our food is producing red things on me which tickle. All my love for always and forever and a day,
Tam

1. Sir Alexander Korda (1893–1956), Hungarian born British film producer.

Margaret to Tam — Two Gates, 4 August 1944

Darling,

The Enos and candles are on their way as soon as I can get some Enos, seems a bit scarce. Please darling do ask me to send anything you want. I adore to feel I can send you something you need, after all what am I sitting here for?

Con spoke to Lou Jackson,[1] I did not get the part, which is a disappointment. However he says there is a smaller part for me, the usual few days, so that is that.[2]

Loo and Prue may come over. I adore having them all about me and feeding them and arranging fun for them. We should have a lot of fun with our family after the war my love. Jimminy how I'm looking forward to it. The plans, the good food to order, the leisure and time to waste and sit and think. And everyday you by me. I do love you so desperately my darling. There could never be anyone else for me ever. Hugo now kisses me twice every time, he thinks it's great fun. He pulls me down and says 'One for Daddy and one for Hugo' and then says 'Now do me'.

The Americans are doing wonderfully well and the news seems pretty good from France altogther. Hope this good or better weather holds. The Italian news seems to be better lately too, they are certainly killing a lot of Germans which is good. Wish I could really know what goes on inside Germany. What do you think, is it a hoax or a put up job as an excuse for a purge or a genuine break? If it is a break or split in the army it must be pretty large I think.

How are you getting on alone my love? Pretty tired I guess. Are you getting someone else I wonder? Alerts all day long here today but have heard nothing.

Goodnight my beloved and God bless you – always and always, your M.

1. Lou Jackson was probably a film producer.
2. The film was called *The Twilight Hour*.
3. The Allies had recently taken Livorno and Ancona, important ports on the West and East coasts of Italy.

Tam to Margaret Normandy, 5 August 1944

My Darling,

A letter from you yesterday about your weekend with the girls. Thank you my love, wonderful of you to love them, not wonderful but sweet and natural. I can always imagine Loo grown up, quiet and elegant and lovely, but Prudie is another matter and all I know of her is that she'll talk her husband's head off.

Had a gala week, everybody flat out. My poor old coder is sort of slap happy and the only idle thing in the patrol is Minnie. While I think of it – if you can get the Allied Expeditionary programme don't miss Combat Diary at 3.30 every afternoon – quite first class and more accurate than anything else and gives you a good picture. Whisky is now an absolute necessity – last night none and I dreamt and fussed about codes and wireless conditions and map references all night which is only from midnight to six anyway. However, I'm not really fearfully tired – it's so bloody interesting and exciting. More when I've more time – I love you so very much and always and always will,

Tam

'A happy marriage is like a long conversation which is much too short.' Maurois[1] – I don't care for epigrams as a rule, they're an effort, but this is good I think.

1. André Maurois (1885–1967), French novelist.

Tam to Margaret Normandy, 12 August 1944

Time was when they called it the Glorious Twelfth on account of the exquisite bird – well it's been a goodish day. Very tired – the move was difficult and my bloody wireless tricky for an hour, which is exactly like getting an engaged ringing when you're trying to telephone a bet which you know will win. Hadn't been here twenty minutes before we added two hens to Minnie – who by the way had a rotten day, she hated the scout car. I hear tonight I may leave A Squadron. Typical. Everytime I see or talk on the telephone to the Colonel he says how well we've done and how very hard we've worked, so of course they have to rearrange.

No more – I would love to my Darling but I'm still busy and I'm tired – I love you my most Beloved Margaret. Always and Always,
Tam

Margaret to Tam Two Gates, 13 August 1944

Well beloved at last I have a moment to sit down and tell you what goes on. Your daughters arrived again on Thursday and left last evening. It is lovely to have them and I adore them but the food problem gets me a bit sometimes, not that it is scarce or anything, but there is just so much per person as you know and when one's family swells so, one's butcher fishmonger etc just will not believe it. However we had a lovely three days.

Thursday was a lovely day and so I took them to the river to swim, had supper and the girls waited up until Gwynne arrived, then they went to bed and Gwynne and I had a drink and a long natter. Money of course had to be gone over and things are coming to a bit of a head. She needs £50 for Prue this term, then there are Loo's fees to be paid too but I don't imagine they will be so much. Prue's school sounds expensive doesn't it? However we had a very friendly chat about it and thank goodness we had a gin in our paws so all is well darling. I really do like Gwynne, she seems so honest and easy to talk to – or I find her so – and golly she is sweet to me. She looked very young and very pretty, but seems very fed up with the play.[1] No money, no houses, but she doesn't seem worried by the buzzy bombs.

Golly there seems to be a ring of Victory in all one reads these days. *No one* believes the European war will last after Christmas and a large number are willing to wager on it being sooner. You and I included, eh Darling? I get quite over excited when I stop quite still sometimes and say to myself – It may only be a matter of weeks before we are together again.

I adore you my best beloved and I feel the same as you have felt lately. It must be the lovely warm weather we have been having and the good news and thoughts of being together again. I lie in bed at night and think and think of you and try to reach you in my thoughts and then pray to dream of you. Of course I never do. Mr Bond or Mumford or some man I've never met appears in my dreams and off I go like any wanton having a wonderful time with them. How can one account for dreams?

It's late beloved so good night and God bless you forever my love. Flints and other odds and ends on their way to you. Also two bottles of whisky.

All my love forever and ever,
Always your own M.

1. Gwynne was appearing in *Quiet Weekend* at Wyndhams Theatre in London from 1941–44. It was the longest running play of the war years.

Tam to Margaret Normandy, 14 August 1944

My Darling,

Wonderful news – if only we can close the gap – but they're good at getting out of trouble. The Campaign is beginning to smell like a Victory – to me with my sensitive nose anyway. Very dirty and rather weary – I have to say to you. I get bored with hearing everyone saying they're tired, so refrain, but to you I say – I'm tired and I need several huge whiskies, a hot bath, a massage, an exquisite dinner and a large clean luxurious bed with you in a small part of it. Have hardly listened to the news or seen a paper – I hope our Russian helpers aren't slacking. Goodnight – my letters are deadly I know – but they're written in a hurry and are only supposed to say I love you, I love Hugo. Take care of yourselves and write to me a lot. Always and Always to you my love,
Tam

Tam to Margaret Normandy, 16 August 1944

My Darling,

Another very hectic day and I heard on the midnight news last night that it was St. Raphael that they landed at – Tout près de la Calanque D'or – Oh la la! Les Moules delicieuses. Very exciting here and the days though actually very long seem to flash by.

No letter from you. Someone told me the other day Warners Studios at Teddington was blitzed – isn't my uniform and great coat there, will you ring up? Suddenly realised today I wasn't smoking my pipe and then realised again it was because I hadn't had time to fill it.

My bad times are between 2 and 4 and from about 10 onwards – Benzadrene is wonderful though. I know my letters are miserable

and disjointed, but I've no time to do better my love. I am well – which is better than a lot of them – and I adore you and we're on the eve of a real old fashioned Victory.
Always and always,
Tam

Tam to Margaret Normandy, 19 August 1944

Well My Darling,

It's been pretty to watch. They really are taking a beating, and the swifter it is and the harder it is the prettier it will be. Very interesting, bloody dusty and exceedingly smelly – mostly cattle. Cows must be killed very easily from Blast – they look like toys knocked over in a shop window with their legs very stiff stuck in the air. Lots of pathetic, tragic sights – wretched little villages. By God it's time the bloody thing stopped.

Wish I could tell you all the news[1] – all we've waited for and worked for and planned and hardly dared hope for is happening before one's eyes. Exactly according to the shooting script – a little ahead of schedule. It's pretty to watch if your favourite colour's khaki. It makes me excited, very, then hungover – then depressed with such endless destruction. Like other things in life – my DAY is divided in two – with halves violently opposed in thought and alternating quite regularly.

I suppose I'd better tell you I adore you – though God wot you'd be lunatic if you didn't realise it. I do, my Pretty. Always and always,
Tam

Missed the post yesterday so I'll add a word. Just had dinner with my neighbours – the best meal I've had to date which I enjoyed enormously until I was told it was the dear little calf that's been under an apple tree in my field for the last week.

1. On 9 August British and Canadian troops launched a new offensive south of Caen. Six days later a massive allied force landed on a hundred-mile coastal strip from Nice to Marseilles.

Tam to Margaret Returning from leave, 22 August 1944

My Darling,

I thought it better to let you sleep and then I had a long look at you and kissed you and by that time I was late – I hated leaving you – it's better in a pub or street – curled up in a warm bed is almost unbearable. No more separations from you – if life will grant that I can fix the wealth and happiness. I feel as always, wonderful though it was, that our days together were dissipated – pissy, I mean frittered away. All I want to do is to be with you. I had the depressions in the aeroplane and decided you didn't love me as much as you used to or nearly as much as I do you. I don't know. Do you?

Goodnight and God bless you my most adored Margaret – each time I see you again I become more in love with you – somehow I don't quite feel such is the case with you. Goodnight my love and God Bless and thank you for everything,
Tam

Margaret to Tam Two Gates, 23 August 1944

Paris has fallen, Oh darling what a prize![1] I knew it last night when I wrote to you, I felt it in my bones. Wonder where you are and what you are doing to celebrate, hope you have some drink my love, but suppose your nose is still to the grindstone and no let up to smack your lips over Paris. The Parisians must be mad with joy tonight – or are they? I can't imagine it at all except in terms of London. Oh if only I could see you or talk to you. But I'm Dorney and baby bound and want to kick over the traces with excitement. Oh well one day you'll tell me my beloved over a bottle, and for this I live. Your return. We are all well and happy. Will write tomorrow again. God bless, I adore you always, M.

1. The Germans lost the Battle of Normandy and by 15 August were streaming back towards the Fatherland. On 25 August the French completed the liberation.

Tam to Margaret Brussels, 24 August 1944

I've just heard the bells of St Pauls on my radio ringing for Paris and Marseilles – and tomorrow or the next day it'll be Lyons and Lille and Amiens, and then Brussels and Rotterdam – Oh my Margaret why aren't we together to share this thrilling splendid feeling, for I know you'll be as excited as I am. From now on we shall be moving I imagine – off again tomorrow at crack of dawn.

Oh golly I wonder how long it will be before I am with you? All the mail and N.A.A.F.I.[1] and everything will go to pieces now I expect with the fast advancing. The Bag[2] is a bit under pressure, and remarked in sulky tones to me the other day – 'It's high time the British Army met some serious opposition and then I can get more sleep.'

Oh, my love, my love, I long for you so much and our life together holds such lovely possibilities. Let's be very careful with it. God bless you my most beloved and treasured,
Always and always,
Tam

1. The Navy Army Air Force Institution provided mobile shops for those on active service.
2. See footnote to letter from Margaret to Tam, 9 July 1944.

Tam to Margaret Belgium, 27 August 1944

My Darling,

I may be going to the more fashionable part of the Continent for the rest of the season. Hoping I shall very much – de luxe travel and plenty of Chesterfields, but nothing about it to anybody yet. Found a four leaf clover a couple of days ago and saw the new moon the same night – 65th of this war.

Later

I'm reckoning in countries now not in capitals, though Paris did excite me only because the French themselves redeemed it. Having pawned it, which they did, they got it out and God bless them. My forecast: Civil War in Germany no definite capitulation, no Armistice might, no sudden lights up – just a gradual though swift cessation of hostilities – this may take six weeks, if there's capitulation complete, any day from now. And it looks like a good year for blackberries. No news yet about my trip which is disappointing, maybe tomorrow. Bloody electric storms interfering with me tonight. My rabbit had a baby which looked like a little baby bird, and I think she's eaten it. Eggs again here and hopes of a bottle of Calvados. Seen some very nasty things left around – very unpleasant indeed and I'm glad I'm not a youth for had I seen them when I was twenty I'd have hated it. Goodnight beloved and I'll see you soon my love and then for always and always,
Tam

Margaret to Tam Two Gates, 30 August 1944

Tam beloved,

The news is coming in so fast and furiously still that one hardly has time to realise one bit of news before the next comes. The prisoner problem must be colossal I imagine, particularly as we are advancing so quickly. I wonder will, or rather can they make a stand and if so where will it be? They seem to have gotten (American?) so disorganised now that the re-organisation will be almost impossible. Oh God I hope they are really and truly smashed this time and on their own soil.

I adore you and like you very much too.

Always, your M.

Margaret to Tam Two Gates, 1 September 1944

My beloved,

Well, Silver arrived this evening rather tired and livid with the railways of England.[1] She is looking very well and as choc full of interest and enthusiasm as ever. It is grand to see her again, she makes me think of you a lot.

Golly the Germans must be wondering how soon they'll be fighting on their own soil, only 50 miles away today and who knows where we'll be by tomorrow's news.[2]

Charles[3] heard 'Ike' talk to the press yesterday – thinks he is terrific with a great charm and personality! What about Field Marshal Monty – he'll be quite uncontrollable now. Should think the flying bombs will soon be at an end, only hope they won't start any other vicious death throes. Well if they do I imagine that can't last long either, Belgium tomorrow

Wonder where you are now my love, do hope you took Minnie with you. Let me know any change of address as soon as you can, I shall be anxious.

I shall give you more news of Silver when I've seen more of her. She was a bit tired tonight I think. God bless and keep you safe my darling, I'm loving you,

Always and always,

Your M.

1. Silver had mislaid all her luggage on the journey (see letter from Tam of 23 November 1944).
2. On 17 August the Russians reached the East Prussian frontier.
3. Their friend Charles Eaton.

Margaret to Tam Two Gates, 4 September 1944

Beloved,

Big and very rushed day. Hugo miles better this morning, hardly any trace of a cold so I decided to let him go after all. He's only over at Burnham[1] and being very well looked after, and I think it will do us all good to be separated for a few days. I was miserable when I came into the house tonight after leaving him there. It seems all wrong not to hear him running about and calling for me. When I was telling him about going he listened very attentively and he said as he was getting into bed 'Want lots of kisses tonight Mummy 'cause you're so lovely and I like your shoes.'

Longing to get a letter from you and hear how you are enjoying your new job and all the bits and pieces. I've had one telling me about the original set up, but I imagine you are far from there by now and well established. I hear from odd parts and people here and there that Phantom have done very well indeed. True? I hope so darling.

Well now the Germans are really getting down to it. They have been told to murder and murder and kill and betray and cheat and lie. In short do any dishonour rather than that we should win. *It won't work,* that *really* is the well-known thin end of the wedge. Once men fight on these terms with these orders, then they are beaten. No self-respect or honour or pride left, therefore they are not men.

Goodnight sweetheart. Be good if you get a chance to be bad, I love you always,

Your M.

1. Joyce, Margaret's home help, took Hugo on holiday for a week to Burnham in Berkshire.

Tam to Margaret Paris, 7 September 1944

My Darling,

It must be a week since I wrote and even now I've got very little time. Had a wonderful day in Paris – a long letter when I've a moment. Am now packed and waiting for a plane for the Midi with my patrol and two jeeps, everybody very jealous. Been waiting all day but weather bad and General High Drama – weather bloody. Should letters be slow or hopeless will send messages.

Always and always, Tam

Tam to Margaret

Paris, attached to 21st Army Group,[1]
8 September 1944

My Darling,

Been fussing and fiddling all day waiting for my aeroplanes, tomorrow early now certain, looks like I go far south and then drive madly north. Have a tremendous letter of introduction on sort of C in C level – the rest of Phantom all certain I'm going straight to the Principality.[2]

Wonderful letters from you my love sounding so much as though you really are fond of me. Soon now my Darling. Peace terms must be going on and mercifully we're refusing everything but unconditional surrender. If two months or six months now means Hugo won't have to waste so much time in the middle of his life, then hurray hurray!

Writing not good tonight (a) I haven't my glasses. (b) We have four cases of captured cognac – marked Wehrmacht. Ha! Ha! Oh Darling, how nostalgic Paris made me, not for Paris – for I shall die with a grudge against that elegant unscarred city with its money-loving people, but for the life that'll begin for us soon now. Those heavenly flashes of luxurious elegance – the scent of bath salts, champagne cocktails, Amour Amour and cigar smoke all clinging to silk sheets, but that's not all. I like that nursery smell too, and the smell of a damp cot, and the smell of petrol dripping from a full tank with suitcases packed and stacked.
God bless – Always and always I adore you,
Tam

1. Tam's unit was attached to 21st Army Group commanded by Montgomery which moved from Normandy eastwards to the River Seine and on to Paris.
2. Monaco.

Margaret to Tam

Two Gates, 12 September 1944

Well my best beloved,

Your letter just after your visit to Paris arrived. Bless your heart, how you must have loved it. Your parcel of perfume for me went off to Richmond[1] and John Fitz[2] wrote this morning to say that as soon as he found a reliable officer he could send the stuff over with he would. He also said he thought it was a parcel most women would give more than their souls for. Darling one, I shall probably continue to smell just of me until you come home and then I shall open the lot and we'll both smell a treat together.

German soil is at last feeling the brunt of battle. Glorious news from all over. The Albert Canal must be their last real try before they return to fight from Germany.[3] I imagine they are fighting quite hard there. Will it go through the winter? I'm afraid so darling. Our next and fifth anniversary should really see the end. I can't imagine it being before. Can you? But I'm sure you'll be home before that and perhaps to stay. Oh God, I hope so beloved. I loathe, detest, abominate – in fact I hate being without you.

Thank you for shopping in Paris for me darling. Wish you'd had hundreds of pounds and been able to get some lovely things for yourself.

The theatre is up and doing again now that the Buzzy Bombs have stopped. But I fear me the list of what is on gives me no yen to dash up and see what goes on. I think I *shall* go up when they do something I'd like to see. Wish you could take me though. For I truly have no one these days darling and my telephone seldom rings. Sad story as Hugo would say.

Good night and God bless you wherever you are,
Always and always, your own M.

1. Phantom's headquarters in Britain was in Richmond, Surrey.
2. J.B.L. Fitzwilliam, a Phantom officer presumably based at Richmond.
3. The Germans attempted to make a stand at the Albert Canal as the allies drove them relentlessly back across France towards Belgium.

Tam to Margaret — The Midi, 16 September 1944

Margaret my Darling,

I seem to have so much to tell you. Can't quite remember where to begin. I think with Paris, which I got to on September 3rd when my job with A Squadron finished. We had to let Minnie go – I really couldn't arrive in a liberated Paris with a gray and white rabbit! We drove in through Versailles and St Cyr, banging and crashing over the pavé in a 15 cwt truck and up the Avenue Kleber into the Etoile, flags and crowds and an atmosphere of en fête, and the whole place lousy with Americans as usual, but there was not the wild enthusiasm I've seen in some of the villages, but I suppose they'd had a week of it and were getting a bit tired. It looked lovely and untouched except for odd burnt out Bosche vehicles, and a certain amount of barbed wire left in straggling disorder, for the Parisians, very short of fuel, had taken all the wooden supports for their fires. A few buildings pock marked from grenades, I imagine. Shop windows a little empty but Fouquet's crowded as I turned into the Avenue George V heading for the Hotel – I left the Patrol outside and went to investigate. I shot a big line and asked for the manager, but every hotel bar the Ritz has been requisitioned by the Yanks and he could do nothing for me except press me to sign the book he'd started of pre-war guests who'd stayed there and were returning. Finally fixed at the Deux Mondes in the Avenue de L'Opéra. We all had a room and a bath each! But no hot water. No electric light anywhere so no theatres, no cinemas, no night clubs, no Spectacles, nothing. So different at night to the gaiety of the streets in the day time. It was heaven to have a real bed again and sleep till ten in the morning and then to the Ritz for a very good hair cut and shampoo (the water brought in in a saucepan) and a manicure, and down to the Ritz bar for champagne. But the whole thing made me long for you so much, and when I walked down the long Arcade with all those entrancing things behind the glass I nearly wept for wanting you.

The French civilian gentlemen are mauve chinned and powdered and clean linened as ever, in, as usual, monstrous suits but looking very new, and the women I suppose were chic, but after not seeing them for so long, and coming from a London of ATS and WAAFS and ladies in their husbands' pinstripes, they looked uncommonly bizarre. Anyway I've never been able to tell the difference between a French lady and a French tart any more than I can tell an enlisted man from an American Colonel – I salute everyone every morning.

There was a scarf in the Ritz I wanted to get for you, but the little girl wanted nearly six quid for it. It had a map of Europe and the Atlantic and America and the English Channel. Across France was written 'La France Libéré – Vive la France'. Across America 'Merci à nos Liberateurs. Vive America'. But north of the English Channel, though space was ample, there was curiously no sign of the United Kingdom. The North Sea merging charmingly with the channel quite uninterrupted by England. Quick work and very French.

I feel I've given you none of the atmosphere. For my own part it was very mixed. What is the good of feeling thoroughly clean and soignée about the head if your shirt smells and your socks are dirty, and what is the use of the dear stuff if you are not at hand? And though pleasant to buy perfumes for you the real pleasure is only if one's pyjamas smell of Amour Amour at eleven the next morning. But God wot it was heaven after ten weeks in that miserable bridgehead in the gray wet windy summer days of smiling Normandy.

The contrasts were strong: parking a filthy truck in the Place

Vendôme, the colour and excitement and gaiety and fun of the day time, and the miserable let down in the evening with nothing to do and nowhere open. Millions of bicycles even Bicycle Taxis. A wretched man pedalling madly with two people sitting in a sort of three ply orange box being towed behind. Le Velo Taxi. Not knowing Paris well or loving it dearly, and most of my memories of it closely connected and somewhat discoloured with hangovers, I had no joy of reunion. Only a certain satisfaction at having got there and a great longing for you. But it was fun and I'm glad I got there early, even so I wasn't sorry to leave, and I left loving London, every inch from the sparrows and the pigeons to the top of St Pauls.

I hope the trippers of the new world flock again to Paris after the war. They'll find it quite unchanged and just the same. London will never be the same ever – and that's just as it should be. Better not to have a single Wren church left than to have added a word like collaborateur to the world's vocabulary.

I'm stodgy, I must shut up. I hope to heavens this bloody campaign finishes when I think it will. Always and always my love to you, and kiss our Hugo for me,
Tam

Tam to Margaret The Midi, 17 September 1944

Well, on leaving Paris I went back to R.H.Q.[1] and was rather busy getting ready. Finally the planes arrived and after a hell of a job getting the jeeps onto them, and oil pressure trouble in the port engine, and God wot else, we got away. I think it's a deadly method of travel. Arriving at Brignoles of course not a sign of anyone I wanted, so into Aix. Now that really was fun. We were the first English they'd seen, and the lights were on, no blackout, and plenty of cafés and bags of stuff. Great evidence of F.F.I.[2] and La Resistance everywhere. Photographs all over the place of Traitors – both men and women – and also of the heroes of the F.F.I. who'd been killed or tortured by the Gestapo. I've heard fearful stories of imaginative torturing. The silly clots had flown me a good two hundred miles too far south. I had a shrewd idea when we left but who am I to argue with Army Group, and anyway why kick at going to Provence? Lovely weather. Bivouaced that night in the hills north of Sisteron and on to Grenoble next morning by eleven – coffee and green chartreuse after a wet drive and a long talk with the café owner. He told me he was in a Prisoner of War cage with

the English in May 1940 after Calais and they sang 'We'll Hang Out the Washing on the Seigfried Line' until the Bosche were hopping mad. And a story of an American dropped near Grenoble and caught. Crucified with both ears cut off and his mouth stuffed with earth. The Bosche before leaving took 160 million Francs out of the Grenoble banks. The war in this part of France seems to have reached unknown heights of cruelty and hatred, and the F.F.I. must have been wonderful, really wonderful. Their guts and courage unlike anything I've heard of anywhere else, and revenge is being very sweet. No S.S. man is taken. Courts sit all the time trying the traitors. More later my love.
Tam

1. Regiment Headquarters.
2. Force Française Interieure.

Tam to Margaret

The Jura, north of Bourg,
18 September 1944

I finally found the Head Quarters I was looking for, and having been checked and questioned and interviewed and listened to and talked to and given many dissertations on Phantom to a great number of American Colonels ignorant of the existence of the regiment, I eventually got set up. I'd built the whole thing up of course, and then immediately we opened a valve blew and I was out of touch which was simply maddening.

A bit lonely here but fun and interesting. Lots of French officers, most of them charming and a little more grown up and civilised than our other allies. I believe France will take years to sort itself out. What a pity those Bourbon counts are such tripe for France needs a king.

Moving on tomorrow, from now till the end will be tiring I fancy, but I'm immensely glad I'm down here – the Vosges and the Black Forest appeal a great deal more than those dull low countries.

First about the house – get something if you can, but if not don't worry. It must be nice for we've waited so long for it. My priorities are exquisite comfort, excellent food and drink, and holidays the moment I don't work. I'm sick and tired of tents and camp beds and French barracks with lavatories in which you stand up, and washing all over in a basin that wouldn't hold a dozen potatoes, and little tiny cottages with the noise of the plug re-echoing down the street, and having to drink in pubs – I wish never to walk further than the sideboard for my drink unless it is to the fridge for more ice.

I'm moving tomorrow, north of Besançon somewhere. I'm doing the normal work here, only I'm alone with the patrol. Getting a little nervous that the high level plan is leisurely and not swift – but if it's annihilation I'm all for it. What's a month if it means Hugo won't ever wear this fearful colour, and Loo and Prue's little sons won't have their lives interrupted? I personally think before November. No more my love except to thank you for being my wife and making the thought of the future quite perfect. I will take care of the happiness. God bless you, be patient, be good, wait for me, I won't be long. Always and always,
Tam

Margaret to Tam — Two Gates, 20 September 1944

Sweetheart,

What a lovely exciting day you have given me today. After a lot of mix up and too many cooks spoiling the broth, the parcel you sent me from Paris arrived. Oh it *is* really beyond description. I feel like a Princess receiving glorious gifts from some far off Prince. Perhaps I am! And all on the same day as the news of your safe arrival. What could be better darling one. I'm so glad you are safe and well wherever you are and now I shall begin to hope for a letter. I've written to all your men's wives and mothers and told them you are all well and safe and if there's anything I can do I shall be most happy etc etc. O.K.?

You *are* clever darling, the scents are too wonderful. Just to open the lovely boxes did me and my morale a power of good. Everything I love, in the scent line, is there. Powder lovely, lipsticks *terrific*, no nails for the varnish but perfect colours so I'll grow my nails if I can. I just *can't* make up my mind which to send Gwynne though. But I'll send one darling, you may be sure.

Just lately I've had a lot of black curtains of depression round my head and shoulders. I can't think why, just perhaps because the days are slipping by and Christmas coming nearer and I can't even dare to hope you will be with us by then. But maybe you will. And then all that lovely scent and no one really gives a damn how I smell. I shall keep it all for you darling I think. God bless you my most precious beloved. Hope you are having an interesting time

still. Take care of yourself and remember I love you always and always, your M.
Hugo's usual damp but loving kiss.

Margaret to Tam   Two Gates, 25 September 1944

Beloved,

Still no news of you, but I am not worried at all as I expect to have to wait quite a little while longer. Anyway I have had news of your arrival so I know you are hard at it again.

Boysie, Vi and Charles' little piano playing friend, has been down with them for the week end and played some lovely old tunes to us last night while we all sat round in heaps and thought our own memories. 'Remind Me of You', 'Always', 'Make Believe', 'Foolish Things', 'Thanks for the Memory', 'All the Things You Are'. I just sat in a big chair with my eyes closed and wanted to shout and shout with the pain and nostalgia to listen gave me. Then when I got to bed I could not sleep for thinking and wanting and remembering. I think the dear stuff gave me ideas – we drank to you and your swift return darling, but it does not taste the same sans you, you know.

A great friend of mine pre-you days, Ian Fenwick, has been killed. Upset me a lot. He was a grand person, very amusing and good looking and a well-loved man. Why do these men always seem to get one? God does take our charmers early, does he not?

Unlike you my love, I still have no hopes of Christmas, never the less you do and this is your home so I'm laying plans.

What do you think I did yesterday? I made up my mind that that poor miserable girl Jacqueline Deniham must be visited and off I went. Surbiton! It took me two hours to get there and same back. But it was worth it. Oh dear, never have I felt or seen such gratitude. Her mother was pathetic and *so* kind. And J was just as I expected – a hideous mess of illness with a simple, sweet, child's mind. Her room is full of you and me, and her life too I fancy. She can never go out unless in a car with her parents and she only goes to see us in films. So I did a thing I should have done for once. I know you'll be glad I went darling.

Gradual annihilation is the plan for Germany Tam, and it's going to take time. They will dig themselves in, in small rotten Hitler-worshipping groups all over the country and our chaps are going to have to dig them all out. Early next year for sure, but I dare not hope before.

Hugo is his usual loving boisterous self and sends kisses to Daddy. I send *all* my love always, your own M.

Margaret to Tam Two Gates, 26 September 1944

Beloved,

Lovely wonderful long letter and short mad one from you this day. So I've had a grand time with maps tracing out your trip. From now on I imagine you'll be pretty 'nose to the g stone'. Aix etc sounded quite fun. Darling it was a wonderful letter, I could imagine it all and it made me *long* to have been with you. And you too, made me wish I had been. By the time you get this I suppose you'll be much further north, probably in the last place you mentioned. Not too close I hope. What really rotten luck about your set, you must have felt very frustrated indeed. Have the Americans made you a Col. yet? Try hard, you know the attitude of the Green Room.

Just had to go upstairs to Hugo. Tears and I finally discovered he had a hair in his mouth, very nasty. He said 'Mummy Hugo's un-set' Always says un-set for upset which I adore. And after I've been cross or smacked him he says – Shall a get (forget) about it now Mummy? He told me yesterday that he thinks he is quite big enough now and is going to wait for Daddy to come home before he gets to be a man. He had a card from you this morning. I read it to him and he just looked at me and took it out of my hand and stuffed it up his jumper and went into the garden. I thought he had forgotten about it. But later I saw him take it out when he was alone and study it hard and long. Funny little chap. Strong loves and dislikes already.

Taking Mum to the movies after lunch so must get cracking. All all my love for ever and always, your own M.

Tam to Margaret Nr Besançon, 26 September 1944

I'm in a curious abode. It rained incessantly for a week and got considerably colder, so I decided tents were no good and have installed the Patrol and myself in a derelict Tramway Halt Shelter affair – the roof leaks and the windows are broken, but there is a kind of stove and it might be worse. The Bosche took the tram lines away for salvage, hence its disuse. The work is tricky rather than hard. Being in an American sector it is fun to be welcomed because one is English, though at first they all thought we were F.F.I. on account of our berets. But in spite of the welcome – the flags – the banners – 'Bienvenu aux notres Liberateurs', 'Merci à nos Allies' and all such, having put up the decorations they hopped inside to put up the prices and having done that they ran downstairs to water the Cognac. There are rare exceptions and last night I dined (very well but almost in the dark, no electricity, no candles, only tiny little wicks on bits of cork which float on oil which in turn floats on water in a tumbler) with a little man I met in a café. His mother, born in 1868, was a charmer – in all she's given a husband, two sons, two sons-in-law and a grandson since 1914 and had herself been hit in an R.A.F. raid on Paris last year. But she's another three sons and twelve other grandchildren and a face that was soft. The stories of torture and cruelty and unbelievable brutality nearly make one sick – really I mean sick – and they are unbelievable except for the force and the faces of the people who tell them. It makes the end of the war, though God knows how one longs for it, seem so unimportant. Nothing, nothing, nothing, not you nor me nor any of us matters, but the complete utter entire destruction of Germany. Bombs, coupons, blackout, restrictions, whiskey at £3, no comfort, no taxis, no real life as we know it – what are they really to being hungry and terrified and on sufferance in your own land with friends and neighbours being burnt and tortured, fingernails and electrocutions and floggings and dreadful things with children that make no sense of anything, any words or meanings we've ever contemplated in our most horrible moments. Shaftesbury Avenue is as far away as the Pole Star. It's most irritating that the sixth year of the war finds me at last with a reason, a motive and a longing to annihilate. But have no fears, all I do is send my little messages as safe as a little mole in the ground. Now I've started to write I long to go on but I'm sitting on my camp bed in acute discomfort with my back breaking and no support anywhere. Send this on to Mum and Gwynne for I have no more time,

Goodnight and God bless you all – I miss you so much,
Tam

P.S. Margaret my darling, A line for you and you alone. I'm missing you and wanting you terribly at the moment. Having no regular mail from you and not knowing how you are is misery and Oh God how I long for it to be all over. But only, as I said in the rest of this letter, if it's really over – never never any more misery and the cruelty and oppression. But that doesn't stop me longing and wanting you and loathing the wet and discomfort more than ever – it's so unpleasant. I haven't been clean or not smelly for three weeks, no, more, since I was in Paris.

Margaret my Pretty, I'm more randy and hot pantsy than I've

ever been in my life. What is it? Is it my swan song? Is it I love you more? Is it the rain and the climate? Is it my age? Is it the end or the beginning, I'm really worried. At night I can't sleep for thinking about you and soon I shall be getting back to the avenage[1] I played with myself when I was fourteen. And what will happen on my return? Oysters and champagne and once a fortnight? But you should be in my tram shelter tonight my Darling.
Always and always,
Tam

1. A word possibly derived from the French 'venir', to come.

Margaret to Tam Two Gates, 28 September 1944

Beloved,

Well thank God Arnhem is over,[1] what a ghastly time those men must have had. However they have done a great job and whatever is said *now*, I'm sure history will tell that their job was well done and worth while. Eight days of hell though it must have been.

As for house hunting, I think your plan is best. Stay here but keep looking, and if you are home for Xmas well and good and perfectly glorious. We'll take a mansion and have a lovely Christmas and then set about finding something for just Mr and Mrs Williams and son. Oh how I long for all our dreams and plans to come true darling, and they will, won't they?

Not much news to tell you today my love, but just so that you shall have your daily scratch from me to remind you that I'm waiting for you and loving you every hour of every day,
Always and always, your own M.

1. As part of a joint Allied operation to gain control of the Lower Rhine the first British Airborne Division was to seize the bridge at Arnhem. The Germans fought back strongly and the venture ended in bloody failure on 25 September.

Tam to Margaret Nr Besançon, 28 September 1944

Had my first hot bath today since June 12th. The Public Baths re-opened in this town, God what a pleasure. I had a couple of cold ones in Paris and a chilly swill in a bidet in Aix, but that's all, apart from sitting in canvas in the open with the breeze blowing and drying the soap on you.

Last night I dined with another chum I picked up in a café.

Four children who all dined with us, Jacques aged five passed out after his glass of wine quite peacefully. He's been in the F.F.I., captured and given the business. They put him in an asbestos room and then heated it way beyond Turkish Bath temperature, and kept him with the sweat pouring off him hour after hour, getting weaker and weaker. Then they'd cold douche him, then more heat. Every half hour he was questioned again. All told quite simply with a sleepy kind of smile. His brother who'd been a Professor at the Sorbonne is now a labourer in sabots and a cropped head in Germany. Oh God, Oh God one's heart nearly burst with pity. Vengeance, vengeance, vengeance – how can they think of anything else?

Oh dear, the Ist Air Borne Division – an error and how![1] Another epic, another page of glorious history has been written. An example to future generations of the British Army, in keeping with the finest traditions – all the old dialogue meaning a cracking, bloody, costly, appalling defeat. How we glory in them. The most famous battles of the last war – Mons, Gallipoli, The Somme – all absolute disasters, and in twenty years we shall be talking of the glories of Dunkirk and the Airborne Landing.[2] Give the dear dear English a disaster and they're happy – and magnificent. A victory brings only embarrassment of having to be diffident and casual about it. And how our lovely language has suffered since the last time our Armies invaded, under Henry V. 'On you noblest English', and his prayer 'Oh God of battles, steel my soldiers' hearts'. Compare them to messages I've seen and passed: 'Bum on.' 'Amiens tonight or bust' and Monty's 'We'll knock them for six.' Hurray for the twentieth century! Bed now my love – dear God when will it be with you my darling? Six winters is really too much. It'll end soon, but I want complete destruction, even if I'm sitting in my tram shelter this time next year. I even think I'd like to kill a German nowadays!

Always and always,

Tam

1. Tam is referring to the British failure to capture the bridge at Arnhem.
2. The British managed to change the public perception of massive defeat in the First World War, at Mons, Gallipoli and the Somme, into moments of glory. Tam fears they will do the same with Arnhem and Dunkirk.

Tam to Margaret Nr Besançon, evening, 28 September 1944

God how I miss you, and how I resent your not being here, for it's such fun in many ways and enormously interesting, and with you here we'd be having such a wonderful time. I wouldn't have missed it for – well, all the boredom and waste of time, and *loss* of time, and loss of money and the discomfort and separation of the last five years seem worth it now.

The principle [*sic*] reason for going to Epsom was always to avoid reading what R.C. Lyle[1] wrote about it in *The Times* the next morning, and to save oneself the irritation of buying a paper at 3.28 from a ruffian running out of an alley screaming 'Derby Winner'. So I feel about the war.

I've been tremendously lucky – very very few people can have seen as much of France in the last three months as I have, certainly nobody in the army, maybe De Gaulle, but no one else much, I reckon. And of course the joy of always knowing exactly what really is going on is worth everything.

The whole Regiment has had such a resoundingly crashing success – originally designed for just two armies, the British and Canadian, we now serve about eight, and that makes one oddly but extremely delighted. It's been fun to watch the success of it down here too, for they'd never heard of us a couple of weeks ago. My Tramway Halt Shelter is getting quite cosy – which of course means we shall be moving soon.

More later my love,
Tam

1. R.C. Lyle was the Racing Correspondent of *The Times*.

Margaret to Tam — Two Gates, 29 September 1944

Beloved,

Wonder just exactly where you are now and what you are doing. It is 11 o'clock (A.M.) here, a dull cold day. Hugo is in the garden and I'm off to Windsor to pick up the fish for lunch.

A lot of numb skulls here are of the opinion that Arnhem was a big failure. Surely it has been a major success except for the great loss of life, which we all loathed to hear and read. *But it was a success*! They did not die in vain. People are odd. One serious and gripping piece of news with a certain loss and not immediate swift advances, and they say the news is bad. I think it is colossally good, but I still can't see Christmas clearly. Can you?

Johnny – oh dear, the menace wants to write to you (Darling Daddy come home soon to Hugo xxxxxxxxxxxxxxxxxxx)[1]
Johnny says he is out of touch with you and will I be go-between. Should he buy a car and keep it over there until we, we meaning

you, can go and fetch it. I said yes, a good idea. What say you? I must fly and I'll love you for always and always,
Your own M.

1. Dictated by Hugo, who added the kisses himself.
2. Johnny suggested he should buy a car in France on Tam and Margaret's behalf, but the plan was never put into action.

Tam to Margaret Nr Besançon, 4 October 1944

My Darling,

A short note by quick way to send you my love and tell you all is well. Missing you very badly, am rather depressed about the War – we're winning of course, but how well the enemy are losing, and I think not this year now. But that surely must be the best sign there is for I've been wrong since Munich.[1] My love to Hugo and all and always my darling,
Tam

1. The Anglo-German Accord signed by Chamberlain and Hitler on 1 September 1938.

Tam to Margaret Nr Besançon, 4 October 1944

My Darling,

Mail from you came today. It filled me with abject nostalgia and longing for you and homesickness and a great surging urge to talk to Hugo.

I feel like you we're in for another six months at least and I'm beginning to feel like Cinderella – I must get home by midnight. Not that my beautiful clothes could have turned into anything much more repulsive than they are at the moment.

Very comfortable now. A young man at this H.Q. greeted me warmly, using the correct Tam as opposed to Hugh. I was charming naturally, but a great deal more so when I discovered he was not only the Requisitioning Officer but also had a bottle of Pernod. With the result that I have a little flat and he has no more Pernod. I have him taped now for the highest available villa whenever we go, so most of the winter's problem is solved. I'll have all the Patrol in beds and off the floor in three or four days.
Always my love, my blessed one,
Tam

Margaret to Tam — Two Gates, 9 October 1944

Beloved,

So far I've had an extremely abortive day. Dashed off to look at a house which was *not* in a village and practically semi-detached. Awful. 7 guineas too.

Papers say Aachen[1] is isolated and they are fighting in the streets, so by now I imagine it will have fallen. Cologne this week! Oh golly I hope so. I wonder if it is getting very cold where you are darling. I read somewhere there was snow on the ground round Belfort. Don't let yourself be cold beloved please, I know how you loathe it. How about a sleeping bag?

Are you being good? Do you love me? Oh Gosh I wish I could be with you, always your own M.

1. On 10 October the Allies surrounded Aachen and forced the Germans to surrender.

Margaret to Tam — Two Gates, 10 October 1944

Darling One,

Lovely day today. Took a bus over to Berkhamsted to see the house agents and see what the position there is re houses. Pretty bad I fear. I started to walk back to the bus and on my way I saw *the* house. Oh darling it was perfect. Of course I did not go in. People definitely living there and how they must love it. A beautiful Georgian farmhouse, the sort of house that makes one think of happy gay weekends, lots of children playing about, plenty of good food and drink and people living in it who are peaceful and good and loving and who like each other. Of big chairs and sofas and masses of books and plenty of music. And good big beds and clean clean sheets smelling of lavender.

Oh darling, we will be able to forget all the times we've been separated and just live with and for each other and being good and happy, won't we? I don't mean to forget all the horrors and the deep vileness of all the Germans' crimes, but to remember and yet forget. I can't quite explain what I mean. But perhaps I mean that we will appreciate all we have more *because* of what has been. I do love you so deeply my darling and I so very much want to make up to you for all you've done so willingly and with never a grumble except of course occasionally to me, which I like because it makes me feel you are close to me, and only say these things to me because you know I'll understand. It has got to be got out of a system otherwise it never heals up. I am gabbing on, aren't I?

Wonder what the Germans will do about Aachen? My bet is they'll fight, the apes. I hope we pulp them! I still say by our next anniversary, wedding I mean, not loving.
God bless you and keep you safe darling,
Always and always, M.

Margaret to Tam Two Gates, 11 October 1944

Beloved,

Well, I gone and been gay today, had a letter from you this morning, lovely and full of news. Yes, I can understand how some of the stories you hear make you feel truly ill. I've heard quite a few now and they make me feel the same. I also agree with you about the end of the war. Golly we are lucky and this being so, surely we can spare a little more time to see everything properly buttoned up. I hope the government don't imagine we can alter the Hun with kindness and gentle hints etc. No one will ever be able to. God the horror of our chap having to go off to another war even more horrible than this one. I'd rather live on a desert island for the rest of my life. In fact we may do this eh darling? Fruit, sun, sea, sand, and you. What more could a girl want?

Your tram shelter sounds pretty bleak darling. Can't you get a few comforts or furniture from the locals? But as you say, the better you get yourself fixed the sooner you'll move for sure.
I love you my husband, for always and always, your own M.

Tam to Margaret Near the Moselle, 11 October 1944

Darling,

The aeroplane which should have taken my yesterday's letter was delayed. So there's another chance to get in a quick one. How passing strange and very sad that the lovely words 'Quick one' should ever be used in such a meaning. Never mind my Pretty – quick ones will come a plenty. What abject fool said that anticipation was better than realisation?

Have you seen Larry's Richard III? Send me any notices you can though I suppose they're dead and gone. I should imagine he's stupendous – he has the right touch of madness and strength and humour.

Time's up, goodbye now. Oh My Darling How I Love You. Wait for me. Anticipation – bollocks.
Always and always,
Tam

Tam to Margaret The Vosges, 15 October 1944

My Darling,
A case of pink Pommery is on its way to you. Before I leave this land I shall return to Rheims for a jereboam [*sic*] for our next meeting. Why one has never been there before I can't imagine. Driving through these immense gates with Pommery and Greno in enormous gold letters over them really made me feel St Peter must be within call. You'll have great trouble with the corks I warn you, they nearly all break and a corkscrew is necessary.

Well, the Colonel has arrived. Dear God what a boring little fellow, full of simple sophistication which is, with the possible exception of bestial cruelty to children, my most disliked of human qualities. However he promised me a change when he thinks this front goes dull and was as usual very complimentary, which is like getting a good notice from a poor critic – valueless for he simply doesn't know the form.

I'm in a black mood, longing for you and missing you and wondering if this bloody war will ever end. We've waited so long. God knows one ought to be flogged for grumbling, for the price paid has been infinitessimal compared to millions and millions, but I get a little concerned sometimes when I think it'll be eight years since I was in a theatre by the time I've finished and God knows what kind of havoc they may have caused. Cashed another forty quid today which brings what I've had up to £65 – fix immediately with Connie.

Goodnight my best beloved. Five years is a long time. Maybe Mr Mason[1] or Mr Clements[2] would have been a more suitable choice.
Always, Tam

1. James Mason.
2. John Clements (1910–88), actor. At the time of writing they were both in England making films, explaining Tam's bitter suggestion that Margaret had made a bad choice.

Margaret to Tam Two Gates, 17 October 1944

Tamèd my Darling,

Lovely letters and parcel from you today. Golly what fun we had reading them. I'm sending you the Polyphotos of Hugo today. I've marked the ones I like and will you do the same darling? I was watching him through the kitchen window this morning and told him not to sit in the wet grass. He came over and said 'I think I'll close the window', which he did. Then thinking I could not see him so well promptly sat down in the grass. He is nuts.

I've been trying to trace your movements from your letters on the map darling. Golly if I'm right you've been a hell of a long way. A lot of it must have been fascinatingly interesting darling. I'm delighted to hear about your flat, but has it no lavatory darling, or do you mean the men?

News is certainly slower these days but I'm not depressed about it. It had to be expected. Oh but if only we'd invaded a month or even two months earlier. Then indeed you might have been home by Christmas. Now I doubt it my love. Unless you can pop home for a day when you go back to 'A'.[1] That is if you do. Yes that would be marvellous darling. There must be some reason you could think up to get them to send you home if only for a few hours. Oh beloved I'm quite excited just thinking of you coming home. I do miss you so desperately – this time I think more than last, perhaps because I feel now that it is all going to be over fairly soon and I want you back to talk to and *plan* with and in our spare time (which will be a lot I hope) we'll beise and beise and beise until neither of us can walk properly. This is bad for me, I must not think! But don't spoil our future darling, leave Jacko alone and I'll take care of him when you bring him back.

God bless you, all of my love darling, always and always,
Your own M.

1. Tam was working in southern France, separated from his squadron. Margaret hoped to see him before he rejoined it.

Margaret to Tam Two Gates, 20 October 1944

Beloved,

I've just had a lovely but faintly upsetting letter from you. You don't seem to be getting my letters at all. So before I tell you how excited I am about the dear stuff I'll answer your questions and put your mind at ease.

Don't worry my darling, I'm in touch with the bank and will do my best to see that the cheques do not bounce. I've asked about the 1/6 a day for Commissioned Officers and they are waiting to let me know within the next few days.

The parcels of sweater, muffler, gloves, wrist warmers, soap, candles, hot bottle etc have been sent off. Your cap has been ordered but will be two weeks before they get one for you, also the extra Devon badge.

How long are my letters taking to reach you sweetheart? I've a feeling you are not getting nearly all of them. Your letters arrive very well, that is, the ones you send by someone. Others take weeks. The one I got today was written on the fifteenth, five days, wonderful. Do take care of your cold. I've been so worried you'd get one and not be warm enough. You are doing a wonderful job my Tamèd and don't ever think you are not. All those young men are also doing a grand job and they are the age for it. You are quite right to admire them but don't envy them darling. You've got a good job, one you can do well. Surely that is as it should be. Anyway I'm as proud as a queen of you and always have been (with one or two possible exceptions!!) and always will be. I suppose as you say one can't choose, I just *had* to have you my beloved, so I married you and I'm glad I did my Tam every hour of every day of every year.

Don't worry darling, Hugo is the only man I sleep with these days. However I can't say I don't think about it, and quite a lot lately. As the evenings get longer I sit in front of the fire and dream day dreams of us being together and making love and plans and more love and playing our gramaphone [*sic*] and drinking. I love all the part of being together, *living* together. I feel I'm too old for just 'Popping' darling, but this is what I want it to be now. I know what my life is to be now and I want so much in the future like you darling, so I shan't muck it up and I hope you won't either. You won't, will you? I'd have gone off long ago if I'd had the misfortune to marry Mr Mason or Mr Clements *and you know it.* Now I think I've answered your letter so I'll tell you what there is to tell about us.

Sorry you are low and depressed sweetheart. 'You and me together love' and take care of that cold.

I've done my three months treatment advised by Dr Maxwell and I shall be going to see him again next week. I'm much more regular now but still about 33 days instead of the usual 28 which is not right. However, perhaps you'll fix that for me when you come home darling!! Oh I wish you could get home if only for long enough to start another baby darling. I do want one so badly. Can't you fix it, oh can't you? Six months sounds like an eternity to me and the war can't possibly finish before the Spring now. Can it? I'm sorry to grumble too my love, but time is slipping by and Hugo is getting so grown up and our next baby will be so much younger than he is. I'm doing my best to get right so that you won't have to try so hard next time darling. I do miss you so terribly but Hugo God bless him is wonderful and makes up for a lot. You could take him anywhere with you now alone. I'd adore to see you both going off together. He suddenly said yesterday 'I do love Daddy' and I said why? And he said 'I just do, that's all.' I know what he means, because I just do too.

This letter is far too long darling. I hope it doesn't tire you out reading it. But I love writing to you, it makes me feel close to you. All my love always and always,
Your own M.

Tam to Margaret — The Vosges, 21 October 1944

News not very startling, the most dramatic even being a cut thumb, caused by a stubborn cork and a couple of inferior cork screws. The result, a considerable quantity of champagne spilt and quite a little blood. These being the two most precious fluids I was naturally incensed.[1]

I've had the black depression heavy on me recently. I believe it's chiefly drink. I think really the 'depression' may be the wrong word and boozies gloom a wrong diagnosis. I think perhaps I'm in love, awfully in love. Or is it a habit after seven years? NO. It's the well-known agony and nothing half so cosy as a habit, damn it. I think '37 must be a rotten year for Pommery, I've never written so horribly before.

God bless and wait for me. In a recent letter you said 'Be good if you get a chance to be bad.' Very ambiguous. I return the injunction to you with the addition 'If you're bad be lousy!' But I'd prefer you to be patient.
Always My Darling Always,
Tam

1. This was the only 'wound' Tam sustained during the war. He cut a tendon and was unable to straighten his thumb again.

Tam to Margaret The Vosges, 22 October 1944

My darling,

I saw my wounded friend off on his aeroplane this afternoon. He's a very young rather charming boy called Peter Johnson. He may telephone you when he's a little better. Be nice to him. He's had a perfectly bloody time and deserves to be spoilt and petted. He's just been telling me his mother had her first son born during the last War and her last, a fellow of Hugo's age, born in this one, which appears to me the most admirable achievement.

Poor little Peter. So young, so frail, so terribly in need of his mother and warmth and kindness and safety. Two days ago when I drove him forty miles to meet the plane and it didn't turn up I was hard put to it to comfort, and my heart went sloppy. I remember Loo's face when she was about eight years old having waited for some farm child for an hour, drifting back to me with disappointment and disillusion – those two old charmers – looking out from those lovely eyes. He seemed to hate the thought of going back to hospital, so I kept him here. Quite right. Three hours and he was in London and the temptation to jump in was almost overpowering. Then back to find the latest arrival from R.H.Q. had arrived but had been given no mail to bring us. God damn their idle lazy bloody little souls – golf and matinées and dinner parties – Christ I'm angry. For five bloody months I've pacified my Patrol with patched up excuses for their unforgiveably careless methods, but I'm beat now. 'No mail Sir?' from four disappointed miserable faces, and mine made an enraged fifth.

Then back here and a lovely row with an old French major at dinner who started saying the Maginot Line[1] must go right up through Holland after the war. God of Love and Tears! I wonder how many people realise that modern war was made old-fashioned on August 6th when rocket firing typhoons shot up 101 German tanks on the road to Avranches? That was a date. The Tank became obsolete in about an hour and thirty minutes – and future warfare is left right open to the scientists.

How I'd been longing for a letter from you and those cosy bastards go and forget it. And to think I sent them a couple of bottles of Pommery and Greno '37, and not a word of acknowledgement. I really am annoyed. My love – again and again and again and as usual on paper – My Love. Hell and Darkness! Damn their carelessness. Goodnight beloved,

Tam

1. The Maginot Line was a system of fortifications built by the French between 1929 and 1936 along their frontier with Germany from Switzerland to Luxembourg.

Margaret to Tam Two Gates, 24 October 1944

Beloved, another lovely letter from you this morning. Bless your heart darling, with all the champagne you didn't sound very cheerful. And I've seldom known champagne to give one the glooms. I think what we both need is to be together again and badly. Oddly enough I've had the glooms a bit lately, but I've put it down to being on the wagon and having the curse. But I'm coming off with a high-class bang for the dear stuff. Do darling take care of your thumb, you are such a duffer with your paws but I did think you knew how to open a bottle without gashing yourself. Golly darling, seven years in Jan – the eighth to be exact. If it is a habit I've got, wanting you, I hope I have it all my life because it is a habit I love and enjoy. They say the first seven years are the worst. But for the times we've been together during the past seven years, I can't imagine being happier or more in love. I love you more now than I did the day I married you. Oh I wish you were coming home, I do. Dear loves and kisses for Daddy Hugo said suddenly, and insisted that I write it.

Have to go to London on Friday to take Prudie to the dentist. I'll bring her back and take her to see Buffalo Bill on the way home. She really is an adorable little girl, so much sweeter, quieter, natural and more thoughtful when she is alone. Hugo is on the bounce and I can't keep my mind on writing and keeping him out of mischief at the same time. Poor Mummy is in bed with what we think is lumbago. Lots and lots of love my darling from your son and all of mine,

Always and always, your own M.

Tam to Margaret The Vosges, 28 October 1944

My Darling,

Within reach and eye of half a dozen P and G,[1] what a set up for a jolly evening, but I've eaten already, dined is a word I only use now if I can induce the old woman in the Restaurant in the town to let me in. The place has been put out of bounds, all restaurants have, and stupid with four years of German treatment she thinks if she defies the letter of the law her house will be burnt and she'll be imprisoned.

The people here are not as warm and friendly as they were further south, and I imagine Alsace will be even worse. They were fairly cosy here with the Bosche and the Mayor told me that two

bad raids in May did not help the feeling of the people for the Allies. No they're quite different here and the admiration one had for them further south, Grenoble and Lyons and all round there, has turned to the old feeling of dislike and contempt. There are parts of it as splendid as anything there is in the world and parts as rotten.
Always, Tam

1. Pommery and Greno champagne.

Tam to Margaret The Vosges, 1 November 1944

The news is picking up and please God now the War will speed along. I believe it will. I wish I could get up to Holland where it's interesting, getting very bored here.

We must find a nice warm house in a year or so and collect and contrive to have our own home with not a sign of anything in it chosen by anyone but us. And Hugo will bring odious little boys to it in the holidays and having brought them he'll take a dislike to them and we shall be left to entertain them. How well I remember doing that. And later he'll bring pretty girls and our hearts will begin to tremble a little as we wonder which one we've got to get rid of and which to add to the family. And every two or three months our souls will revolt against such domestic respectability and we'll fly to Paris and behave disgracefully.

I've grown a moustache again by the way, still black by Golly. A sure sign of boredom, or maybe a sub-conscious desire to look as un-American as possible. The inevitable happened the other evening when a young man started shooting off his mouth about America saving Europe, and I suppose it'll go on in bars and ships and parties until I'm too old and deaf to hear what the bastards say. But as long as I do hear there'll be rows, damn their ignorance.

This letter must end my love. Tell Hugo to stay exactly as he is till I get back. Not to grow or develop or learn any new words or taste any new tastes. Now is the lovely age and I must love him through it in order to fortify my affection for the terrible years of dirty hands and revolting pockets, the ghastly vocabulary and the abounding faith in Clyde major, and the conviction that both parents are old and stupid and not for public appearance, and I expect too the agony of shame that stage and screen will shed upon him. Oh Dear! What a very great deal we've got to go through my

Darling. I love you very greatly more and more each month and year, so that I look back with amazement at how I thoroughly disliked you in the Spring of '39. My Love, My Love, My Love, I miss you so much.
Always for always,
Tam

Tam to Margaret The Vosges, 4 November 1944

My Darling, My Darling,

Another week nearly over and another letter to begin, but what to say except I love you and I miss you. Maybe there'll be some mail in from you this evening.

Tell Hugo from me he's a mug if he doesn't wear red shoes for as long as he can. Black and brown are the colours for grown up slaves who get shoved around and pushed about. Red for Freedom. And Fun. And tell him a year from tomorrow November 5th I'll make a great enormous thing with a turnip face, with hollow eyes in which burn two bright candles, and its body will be clothed all in khaki and on its head a service cap from Herbert Johnson's and all around him there'll be everything which connects me with the Army. We'll light him and burn him and have fireworks. And maybe one more thumb will go to the devil. Thanks for being so sympathetic. This one's completely cattled. Healed alright, but the tendon must have gone and there's no movement.

Oh my Darling what a difference your letters make. You said it was worse this time, much much worse in every way. Let's sit in the rain with our feet in the Thames, just so as we're together. Let's have a honeymoon in a Tube lift as long as I can look at you. I love you my Darling so very much. And if we're both as much in love with each other as we say we are – I am, are you? – then by God we've brought off the Great, the Grand, the Biggest Coup in Life and if you died tomorrow or I was killed tonight it wouldn't matter for we've had it, not quite fulfilled it yet, but we've touched all round it and Oh! my Darling it has been sweet. Nothing seems in focus when I'm not with you and my mind takes on a kind of doziness – like an anaesthetic to help me through till there you are.

Beloved this is an appallingly bad love letter. I hadn't meant to write a love letter. I'd have to be a lovely poet, and who in all the history of the world loved anyone as rare as you? How much easier it is for you to get to Brussels than for me to get home. Come to Brussels. People are coming there I know. To hell with Hugo,

come to Belgium for Christmas. I'll be there to meet you if I have to swim the Moselle and the Meuse to reach you. We'd get in my jeep and drive for Rheims. My jeep I have had covered in, out of an old tent and some cases of Pommery so you wouldn't be terribly cold. At Rheims we'd pick up two or three cases, one for our own consumption, two perhaps for barter in Paris. I could fix a flat there, but it wouldn't matter, we could put up a tent in the Etoile and make love until it was time to go to the Ritz for a bath. I mean all of this idea. They can't cashier you. Come on. Be Australian for once, only for once. I adore the sight and the sound and the scent and the touch of you. Bring them to me.
Always, always,
Tam

Tam to Margaret The Vosges, 5 November 1944

My Beloved,
I suppose my letter last night was cock and it was absurd to imagine you could get to Brussels. You're too valuable where you are, so pay no regard to it. Thank you my Darling for the letters. I shall read them again tonight. God bless you my Sweet. I love you. I adore you and always always shall,
Tam

P.S. Let me know when and if the Pommery arrives – I hope those sods haven't drunk it.

Margaret to Tam Two Gates, 8 November 1944

My Beloved,
What really enchanting letters you do write, a lovely long one from you this morning. Full of you and bits to make me laugh and fondness and interest. You started off by saying you had six bottles of P.G. in front of you, but your so-called dinner behind you. What a really bloody arrangement darling. Surely you could 'fix' the old girl at the cafe – get an interpreter darling I always said your French was bad! She probably thought it was an establishment de joi. I just hate to think of you drinking all that champagne alone darling. How I wish I could be with you, and how we'd laugh and plan.

I don't agree with you about the French at all Tam. Yes we've been their Christmas dinner for far too long, but that is our, not their fault and of course their clothes are abominable to us and they are money grubbers. But when all is said and done the blame is on us. There are certain types of English men who are torture abroad and these men and their women and the Americans have made them grab our money. And my golly they certainly do know how to enjoy themselves sans effort. There is a great deal I love about France and the French and with a King I believe it could be the happiest, gayest, most luxurious country in the world. I will discuss this at length darling when I see you over several bottles.

You are right about having a home and Hugo being English but *please* can I go away and get warm in Jan and Feb please. Hugo is outside at the moment making the back garden hideous with old rags, sticks, stones, papers and smashed toys. He treats me as an absolute contemporary. I had a bath with him last night, great fun and splashings. In the middle of it all he said 'Will we bath Daddy too when he comes home?' Oh yes, I said and this seemed to please him. By the way don't let me catch you with that moustache black or white!!! Yes, F.D.R.[1] will get in again. He is determined to die with his boots on. Winston too!

In all we are all well darling and doing nothing very odd or amusing. Just marking time waiting for you to come and get us. I wanted to answer your letter right away as I did not write last night.

My love my love I adore you always and always,
Your M.

1. Franklin Delano Roosevelt (1882–1945), American President from 1932 to his death.

Tam to Margaret — The Vosges, 9 November

My Darling,

Suddenly out of the snow and wind and sleet came letters from you. I've shaken of my black depression. Damn it I really think it was the dear champagne, and have settled down to the winter and the dull routine of dividing the day and night into eating and sleeping and reading and doing the absurdly little work I have. I am warm, thank God, at the moment, for I have my hot water bottle and we went out and found stoves in blitzed houses which my dear little man Robinson has made to function though they smoke a little. The weather is appalling and I think really that is what shook me out of my depression. I suddenly realised how ghastly fox holes must be. I went to look, and never again, even if it comes back, will I dare to tell you. Anybody who sleeps not even in a bed, but just where it's dry, should feel so bloody thankful and almost a shit.

I've been thinking more and more about our domestic future. We've got to buy a house. I'm forty and it's time everything I did was sensible and clean and not stupid and extravagant. I'm not going to live in America because I'd sooner stay in the Vosges than ever hear Hugo call me Pop. Does your heart sink at the thought of a life in England? Not all the time my love. I'm going to have a barge and a very large fast motor car. But however hard I try, when I come back, to spend money, you must stop me. I'm family conscious and worried. No more ridiculous frittering our money away in restaurants, bars and nightclubs (God how I love them).

My favourite tune at this wintry moment is – 'I'll be seeing you in all the old familiar places – my heart – no loving nothing till my baby comes home.' The river swells, the bridge creaks and has a sag in it, if it goes I'm fucked. Tell Hugo how he's complicated our life and thank him for his postcard and the first hot bath I share won't be with him.

Always my Darling, always,
Tam

Margaret to Tam Two Gates, 12 November 1944

Oh Beloved,

What a busy Friday and Saturday I've had. Your letter about Brussels arrived on Friday morning and so I completely ignored the second one saying not to come and immediately went to London. I've set the wheels turning. I've been in a jittering state of excitement every minute of every hour since I read your letter. I rang E.N.S.A. and went to see Stanley Bell and he took me up to give my name and particulars etc. Blond, blue eyes, 5′ 6½″, played Broadway!!!! Toured America!!!!!! Films etc. Apparently Bell only attends to the R.A.F. needs now but he put me on the right track. I then went to see Hartnell[1] to see if he had any plans for Paris or Brussels, he was away but will ring me on Monday. In other words I've put the idea in strong motion and something should happen this week. Oh God I hope so darling. Imagine how wonderful it would be. To walk along a platform towards each other again. Or meet in a bar again. Or jump into a taxi and find you sitting there with a flower for me again. Or be shown into a hotel room to wait for you again. Oh darling it is worth anything. I love you so my best beloved. And I'll *move* heaven and earth to get there. And tell me, will you be fairly mobile because I may not be if I come in a job you know. I told Hugo I might not be with him for Christmas as a strict secret. I said I may be going to see you and he said he would come too. And when I said that would not be possible his little lip dropped and I had a tricky moment. He seemed happier when I told him *you'd* said he must stay and mind the house though. I'll say goodnight now darling and perhaps I'll add to this in the morning if I get any news before the post goes.

I love you my darling always and always your M.

1. Norman Hartnell, couturier, for whom Margaret worked as a model.

Margaret to Tam — Two Gates, 13 November 1944

Beloved,

Being the 13th I truly thought someone would ring up with some sort of good news, for it is usually a lucky day for me, but not a sound all day from anyone. However it is too early to despair. Norman Hartnell may be taking a sort of puppet show of dolls dresses in the various costumes of the Allies in a couple of months – too late – however he did say that if anything came up or there were any chance of his going to France or Belgium of course he'd let me know. I could ask no more. And he asked tenderly after you darling.

Tamèd I do hope you are not drinking too much of the dear stuff or any other stuff. I've had an impression from your letters that you were 'on it' a bit. Now don't be cross, I want you to get all the fun you can out of your drab existence darling and I may be quite wrong. Oh the hell with it, why should I even think you are, it was just an idea my love, forget it.

I've told the little chap about the red shoes and he says then he'll get you a pair of red too when you come home. Good idea, let us all wear red shoes and be free.

I love you and I'll get to you if I have to go to the King.

My darling one I long for you always and always,

All my love,

Your own M.

Margaret to Tam — Two Gates, 15 November 1944

Beloved,

Oh dear, each day that goes by and I have to write and tell you that I have no news about my trip makes me more miserable. Oh I wonder will it come off? Tomorrow I have to ring Connie again and then maybe something will happen. Oh my darling just to think about seeing you and being with you again makes me realise how terribly much I miss you. More, much more than ever before beloved. Oh darling I *do* hope I don't fail, it will break my heart if I have to sit here and have another family (incomplete) Christmas sans Tamèd.

I wonder whether you are warm now darling and are you getting all your parcels?

Funny how tactful the British Press *managed* to be during the American election and then they all turn round and say 'We told you so'. Told us what? S.F.A.!![1] And now De Gaulle for Moscow.[2] Ye Gods *what* will occur there I'd like to know.

People have completely relaxed here and no one even *mentions* when they think the war will be over, unless it's to say very vaguely 'Sometime next summer'. Yes!

I love you very very dearly my beloved so take care of yourself. By the way I'm upset about your thumb darling. See a doctor, get home for an operation if necessary, *thumbs are important*.

All my love always and always,
Your own M.

1. Sweet Fuck All.
2. De Gaulle had gone to Moscow for talks with Stalin.

Margaret to Tam — Staying with Jasmine Bligh, 23 November 1944

Oh my beloved,

How badly I've neglected you this week, but an awful lot has happened, and yet it will not take an awful lot of space to tell you. I wrote to you last on Monday night and on Tuesday Jasmine rang to say Sandy[1] had been killed. Of course I packed immediately and came here. I've heard about broken hearts, but this time I've really seen one. There is no more to say. Whatever Jas has been in the past, she loved Sandy, really loved, adored and was in love with him. And he felt the same about her. Poor darling, she is truly heart broken. It is hard to see someone you love go through the hoop like this, and know there is so little one can do about it except talk talk talk when necessary, listen listen listen when needs be and drink continually, even when the thought of a drink turns your tummy over, just to keep company. Write a nice letter to her darling please. Sandy was blown up by a mine in a jeep on the 10th November, she only heard on the 21st. The fact that she did not *know* he was dead upsets her badly too.

Went for an interview about a job in Brussels. It is for an assistant entertainment officer for a rest club (S.H.A.E.F.)[2] for men, not officers, in Brussels. I would have to sign on for six months. How could I leave Hugo for six months people say. I say I've not seen *you* for five months now and nearly a year last time. I gather it is hard work but if you say the word I 'm almost certain I can get to either Brussels or Paris by Xmas. Which shall it be beloved? Answer me *quickly*. I love you. I worship you. I need you. I must see you my darling if I can. As far as E.N.S.A. is concerned nothing much has happened and I feel that if I wait for that I'll wait until well into the New Year.

Oh how I pray you'll say come on darling, and that you'll feel reasonably sure we'll see each other. I do love you so much my beloved.

Perhaps I can buy your Xmas present in Brussels. What do you want, a daughter?
You shall have it or her or perhaps him.
Always and always your own M.

1. General John 'Sandy' Lane, a young Canadian with whom Jasmine was in love.
2. Supreme Headquarters Allied Expeditionary Force.

Tam to Margaret — The Vosges, 23 November 1944

My Darling and Beloved Margaret,

I foresee the most spectacular fuck up since Romeo, thinking Juliet dead, kills himself in the friar's cell and falls across her prostrate body. Your letter arrived and you have apparently set the wheels in motion for your arrival here. I on the other hand, have started a forlorn hope in progress, to come to England. It is now obviously only a matter of time before I arrive at Claridges, telephone Burnham 582 and discover you're in Brussels. If this sounds as though I don't want you to come or am not longing to see you and touch you and talk for endless hours to you then I'm giving you just as wrong and ridiculous an impression as I did recently when you thought I was drinking too much. You can't send really important messages when you're pissed and you can't get pissed with any decent regularity on £18 a month and present French prices. I had ten days high delight on the S.A.S. operational funds with Pommery but that was all my love.

But let me tell you my news. It is now laid down that all British people with the Army H.Q. (only a score anyway) are entitled to 7 days leave in England. Anyway a dear old Colonel, to whom I once in a moment of generosity and considerable forethought gave a couple of bottles of Champagne, and who commands the British personnel here, sent for me today and inquired when I wished to take my leave! I explained that most regrettably I was not under his command and could take no leave, whereupon he suggested that I write to my Colonel asking for a relief officer to be sent here for a week and he will guarantee me air transport both ways. Now this my Darling is a very very long shot and but for the fact I heard tonight of your intended advent here and I hate surprises almost as much as disappointments, I don't think I would have mentioned it. Now forget all about it. Give my dinner jacket a brush and see I've some clean shirts and don't go far without leaving your telephone number and forget all about it. And don't tell Hugo or anybody else.

Always,
Tam

Continued

Effort to get news quickly reported from here is nearly driving me nuts and I am curious, in quite an abstract outside sort of way, to discover just how long my patience is going to last. The endless deadly bonhomie and wisecracking goodwill is wearing very thin and there is fearful danger of a sudden outburst of very English invective. It bloody nearly came yesterday when some uncouth clod in a effort at a compliment said 'You're certainly not like any other Britisher I ever met.' Added to which I've been sending some sharpish kind of messages to the Colonel who listens to the news and then sends me signals saying 'B.B.C. state so and so can you confirm?' So I replied, 'Cannot contradict, confirm nor compete with B.B.C.' Realising I was annoyed he wrote me a very poor little four line verse to which I sent this answer,

Facts I lack Sir
To send back Sir
But report the truth.
B.B.C. Sir
N.B.G.[1] Sir
Liars too forsooth.
Their reports Sir
Nothing short Sir
Of a lucky guess.
Pay no heed Sir
What you read Sir
In the daily press.

If that sort of thing appeals to the dull little man maybe he'll grant my leave, but I doubt it. My Darling I have suffered so much in silence and been denied so long now the glorious prerogative of answering back, that I plan to be exceedingly truculent when the war is over, which will inevitably include being rude to waiters in very public places.

I decided I really must have another go at writing so I've been hard at it for the last couple of weeks and have produced some twelve to fifteen thousand words. Whether they're in any way entertaining I have no idea. But it makes the time slip by wonderfully quickly and I suppose it's good practice. If only I could spell and had an elementary knowledge of English grammar, and subject matter of general interest to subscribers, I believe I could produce a rather slim and boring little volume, which at best might give Hugo some idea of what I'm like and what I feel and think. (The girls I fear would be shocked.) This anyway is a good enough reason for continuing it. And lacking any kind of stimulating conversation it gives one a sort of mental ENOS which has cured my miserable depression. But I'm no match for my mother. I really think her courage and spirit, when you look back on her life, particularly recently, are simply stupendous. Six years ago she was living at the rate of ten thousand a year in warm sunny California with a husband she adored, to make the transition from that to being a lonely old widow in rooms in Cheltenham through an English winter, War time, having lost all her clothes on the Great Western Railway and with no one to talk to but a little girl of thirteen[2] and to preserve the same spirit and interest in life is something that makes me so proud of her I want to cry. Of course she'll irritate me to distraction as soon as we meet. If only she were old all the time I could get organised and make allowances, but it's these damned intervals when she's younger than you or anybody else I know and as modern in mind and thought as an undergraduate, that fox me into argument and disagreement.

Had a strange message from Johnny Hannay saying 'Splendid news your coming back to us but bring pâte from Strasbourg.' Naturally I shall bring pâté from Strasbourg, why did we capture the Godamm place? But what it means I've no idea.

God bless and goodnight and I'm so fond of you.

Tam

1. No Bloody Good.
2. Loo was living with Silver while attending Cheltenham Ladies' College.

Margaret to Tam Staying with Jasmine, 25 November 1944

Darling darling,

I'm still determined to come to you in Belgium if I can – so look out, beware, make plans *in case* it works. But also my love don't be disappointed if it does not come off. I hope you have written by now, telling me if it must be Belgium or if Paris would do, and how much we shall see of each other etc. I'm dead serious. I wonder were you. Oh darling love, even if it doesn't come off I'll have had a little happiness thinking about it and trying to plan it. The only thing I do worry about is your being terribly disappointed if I can't make it. But darling, whatever happens we'll know we'll be together one day not too far off, forever and always.

From what I can gather from the papers, (they'd hate to think I'd gathered anything I know), the day goes rather well at the moment. How must the Germans feel now? With the Allies closing in on their very heart from all directions and their fake god A. Hitler either flown or lying sick with *yellow* sickness or insanity. They must know it will end against them, and soon, soon darling. I pray it will all be over soon.

I've had a bottle of champagne and 4 gins so I think I must go to bed now. I love you always, your M.

Margaret to Tam Two Gates, 28 November 1944

Darling Heart,

A lovely long letter from you waiting for me last night when I got home. Golly how I needed a letter from you too. Jas and her maid Jane had a blazing row on Sunday night (we were all set to leave and come back here on Monday in time for tea) which resulted in Jane breaking a cup against Jasmine's face in front of the children and then screaming off down the drive to the police. The police arrived and Jane packed and left. That was that. Hugo very upset at seeing the row but I told him it was a game and now he keeps asking me to play the game with the cup. Oh dear, poor little chap went quite white in the face and remained so all day. Jas is still in a daze because of Sandy, and seems unable to act or think for herself, poor old girl.

You sound so optimistic about the war darling, and here am I about to sign on for a job in Brussels for 6 months. Golly I 'd be in a mess if you got home and I was sitting abroad somewhere looking for you. I'm getting very worried and longing to get a letter from you. There is another chance I may get a less binding job in Paris, how about that? E.N.S.A. still silent about claiming my talents!!

By the way I've sent you off the Sunday papers. All the *Henry V* notices. Very mixed in their opinion but full of praise for Larry and the rest of the cast. It can't ever make any money I shouldn't think, let alone pay for itself!

Have you got your hat or your pips yet darling?

Darling I hate repeat hate you with a moustache and you know I do – why deliberately thwart me when I can't be looking? Now take it off and don't let me catch you in it or *I'll* beat *you*.

God bless you and take care of you my beloved Tamèd,
Always and for always,
Your M.

At this time Tam was evidently successful in arranging leave for a week in England.

Margaret to Tam Claridges Hotel, 9 December 1944

Just one more note before leaving our room beloved. No, there is no more hope of your not having gone. I've wandered round and round the room and bath room missing you, thinking of things I'd like to have told you, loving you and wanting you to come back again so desperately darling. The room looks so oddly bare and empty for a room we've been in. There are no signs of your having been here at all. No shaving things in the bath room, no unfolded pyjamas, no nail brush or hair brushes, no C.A.R. bottle. It is empty of any sign of you, not even a Craven A butt. Makes me feel as if the whole thing has been a wonderful dream darling.

I feel much better in the tummy now but my heart is so *lonely* for you already darling. Take care of yourself and be good please and I will too.

All of my love always darlingest,
Your M.

Tam to Margaret France, 15 December 1944

My darling,

This should reach you sometime around Christmas Day for the mails at the moment are bloody. So my Darling have a happy day and keep remembering the whole time that this one really is the last and that next year we'll be together, to do Hugo's stocking and put up the holly and split a bottle in the process and share his onslaught at first light upon our hangovers. I shall be thinking of you all day and missing you and longing for you.

People rather pessimistic about the duration, but I still think three or four months. The Russians are getting near to Vienna and the end will come from there, I hope, I hope. I'm a bit concerned about this leave business, I rather feel my clever work in getting back last week may prove a handicap, but maybe it'll be alright. It's a doubtful blessing anyway, for missing you becomes so much worse after it. I read in the paper this morning the sentence 'During the early years of the War'. It made me suddenly aware of how bloody it has been, I don't mean for everybody, the Blitz and starving Europe and all that, I mean for you and I. Such valuable precious years. We'll make up for them though.

More tomorrow my Darling, God Bless you. I love and adore you and I always shall – always.
Tam

Tam to Margaret Belgium, 21 December 1944

My Darling,

Things as you have no doubt read have taken quite a turn and I've been busier the last few days than I have since the Bridgehead in Normandy,[1] very varied opinions and considerable flap. What should we have done in the last five years if we hadn't both been sublime optimists?

Amongst other things I left at Two Gates was my revolver. I don't quite know what to do about it. Keep it for the time being. The last time it was out of its holster was to crack nuts with in Italy and I broke the stock. I met a man the other night, a most amusing old cosy who told me he drew his in some back alley in Brussels and a lot of aspirin fell out of the barrel!

The Americans have fought splendidly the last week and it all looks very interesting. By the time you see Johnny we shall know a lot more. He still takes too much phensic and is very blotchy. He's probably told you in his letter how we pulled a very dull Colonel's leg into believing I was an airborne Padre! He has the gift of a living and told Johnny later I was just the type he'd like to have there after the War!

Tonight is the longest night and in a month the days will begin to lengthen and the back of the winter will be broken. The Spring will be in sight and maybe the War will be over.

I wish I'd been in the wonderful early days of Brussels, no, I don't. For as far as I can gather there's not an officer or man in the Sqn who didn't have a jump and I like being faithful to you, if you're good I do. If I find you out I shan't bother. But I adore you my darling. God Bless, always, Tam

1. Initial invasion of Normandy.

Tam to Margaret Brussels, 31 December 1944

Darling,

New Year's Eve. I suppose the war really will end in '45, everything seems so slow nowadays. Everyone's tired and worn out. I have dreadful moments of wondering if it will. Winter and war, they're really too much together. How the poor bloody infantry keep going in this kind of weather I can't imagine. God it must be awful. Tonight I shall drink to you and pray the end is near. I know the ending of things is always hardest to take – I'm finding it worse now than at any time since the beginning. Had a very amusing letter from Wilfred[1], discharged from the army as being 'Prematurely old'. A rather bitter letter, I can't really think why for he's in a play and has made a success. Did you read the article in the Express about E.N.S.A.? Five hundred artistes promised for the British Liberation Army by Christmas and there are at the moment only 130. With every theatre in London crammed and booming it's to hell with the Troops and lets make some more money. It's monstrous that actors, deferred as key men, should only be made to do six weeks a year for E.N.S.A. I shan't be able to speak to the bastards, unless maybe to tell them what I think of them.

A Happy New Year my Darling Margaret. 1945 will bring us together and life will start all over again and whether it's rough or smooth won't matter for we shall have each other and so it will be sweet. Then and only then shall we dare to say how unutterably bloody these separations have been. All my love to you for always and always to keep you mine and make you happy,
Tam

1. Wilfrid Hyde-White.

Margaret to Tam — Two Gates, 1 January 1945

Well my beloved,

1945 is upon us, and God willing sometime during the year we will meet knowing that we do not have to part ever again. I had quite fun and a lot to drink but the best party with the maximum of drink and the nicest people these days seems rather flat. The better the party the more I miss you, and I so love to dress up and look pretty for you. And for me to be able to look across the room and see you and know that we shall go home together presently is still thrilling and lovely to me. All these parts of being married I've missed for so long, to say nothing of just having you near in all the ordinary little things that make up a day in the lives of two people who love each other.

I thought of you on New Year's Eve and remembered the day seven years ago. *Of course* I remember you asking me to join you for a drink. But how was I to know it would be Champagne? I'd have come of course. But I agree with you, you wasted eight days that might have been even better spent than they were. A bit slow off the mark you were then Darling. Imagine taking eight days to seduce me!! I knew you'd want to marry me so I could afford to wait. But you might have lost me in New York so easily. And *how* you worked at persuading me to stay at the Gotham with you. Oh well, it was all lovely and great fun and you are still the most attractive man I know, and I love you too, more than I'll ever be able to tell you my darling.

Your parcels for Hugo arrived yesterday afternoon. Golly what a lovely train, and beautifully made too, compared with English toys. More tomorrow my love, take great care of yourself and remember I love you forever and always,
Your very own M.

Margaret to Tam Two Gates, 5 January 1945

Tamèd my darling,

Had two letters this morning, one from you dated Dec 31st, and one from Johnny dated Jan 1st, both very interesting indeed. Your letter sounding rather low and depressed and with very obvious signs of your intentions to get pie-eyed, and full of doubts about the contest ending in '45.

Then Johnny's written the next day, full of false phensic fitness and fun, telling me two lovelies escaped his clutches (I suppose he got affectionate and sentimental). He then goes on to tell me how your landlord found you asleep with an aspidistra at the foot of the stairs. I don't think Johnny made it up, for I know you, and your letter was full of signs of an impending Piss Up. I'd have got you up those stairs my love!! Oh well, I hope you had fun before you forgot, my love, and I also hope you have got rid of your hangover by now. Have you heard about the little pink elephant who went into his pet pub and in silent and sad enquiry put his two little feet on the bar and looked up at the bar maid. She shook her head and said kindly 'No dear, he has not come in yet.'

Sorry I did not write yesterday darling but I was in bed all day with this rotten cold. The news is still, as I read it, very depressing. The battle must be extremely fierce and God alone knows how those wonderful men of ours carry on in this unbelievable cold. I wonder do they ever feel warm. The fact that the promised British Liberation Army leave still continues gives me fresh hope and confidence, but then I suppose that is what it is meant to do.

E.N.S.A. make my blood boil so don't even talk to me about them. But please let me be there when you tell them exactly what you think of them. *PLEASE*. I'm not bad to look at and I could entertain them in my way and I *did* go and say I'd go out for Xmas but not a word have I heard. Bone bloody idle. Wonder what Wilfred has to be bitter about. He lives in comfort and for free with a rich and fairly merry woman. He sees his son when he wishes, he is still in the theatre *and* a success. And he is still wearing clothes he has chosen himself, not a uniform the Government have told him to. I think he's a lucky man. As for him being 'prematurely old', well he was born that surely!

Like you I sometimes wonder what this year will bring. Will it see the end, I wonder? Or will next Christmas still find us praying and longing for some miracle.

All my love my darling, always your own M.

Tam to Margaret

Jan 8th 1938 – Jan 8th 1945
New York – Belgium

Two single words are all I find
For seven years to say of you;
All others seeming to my mind
To matter not: Save but these precious two –
Lovely and Kind

Margaret to Tam — Two Gates, 10 January 1945

Tamèd my darling,

Came back late last night from London having had a lovely time and don't tell Johnny but I saw Sid Field.[1] Golly how I laughed darling and how I wished you'd been with me to see him and laugh with me. But he'll still be there when you come back darling.

Thank God the news is perking up. I was really worried for a bit and felt I was not being told the truth (when I say 'I' I mean the Great B.P.) But it seems that no one was ever really at all worried, in fact it was a good thing and would end it all sooner. I give up. Because Runstedt[2] really looked like getting away with it for a while. Anyway, I am optimistic again thank God.

To return to Sid Field's matinée I had tea and a long natter with Jas who seems quite unable to pull herself together yet, but miles better all the same. Lovely evening, Hermione Gingold[3] came in after the show, she *must* be the ugliest woman in England! But really rather a nice old thing I thought.

No more now darling, must get on with the house. It is *so* wet and slushy out in between snow falls that Hugo can't stay out alone all morning. So I have to go out and play snowballs with him for a bit. Gosh it is cold.

Take care of yourself my beloved and keep warm,
All my love always, your own M.

1. Sid Field, comic actor, died 1950.
2. German Field Marshall C.R.G. Runstedt, Commander in Chief West, led the defence of the Allied invasion of Normandy.
3. English actress (1897–1987).

Margaret to Tam Two Gates, Sunday, (undated) 1945

My Beloved,

So sorry not to have been here when you telephoned last night, but I had been digging all day in the garden with old Johnny, so we were exhausted, hungry and rather cross by the evening. So in no mood to cook we went to Windsor for dinner.

Darling isn't it wonderful about the film!!! And £30 a day, better than ever before. God knows what the film will be like though.[1] Filth I should think! However, 'je mon fiche' [*sic*]. Off to London early tomorrow. Hope you do get back on Wednesday darling, longing to see you and missing you badly already. Anyway, THURSDAY? We shall have a lovely ten days my love. Take care of yourself and remember I love you, Your own M.

1. The deal must have fallen through as Margaret didn't make a film in 1945.

Tam did have a few days' leave, but they were evidently less happy than they might have been. At this point in the war he and Margaret had been apart for five and a half years and the following letters show that the strain was beginning to tell. Tam was unable to curb his suspicions that Margaret had been unfaithful to him and she could not convince him otherwise.

Tam to Margaret Belgium, 28 January 1945

My Darling,

The hours of the journey included the coldest nights in the Straights for fifty years, fifteen hours wait in Calais in a hut and a hangover, twelve in a train without heat, and a rock cake for breakfast the following morning. My whisky saved both my life and reason. Thank you. Goodnight to you my beloved, my love always, Tam

Margaret to Tam — Two Gates, 30 January 1945

My darling,

Was there ever I wonder a more tricky letter for me to write? But whatever happens I'm not going to tear this one up. Anyhow I suppose I'm just being silly really, but you said that my letters were more in love than *I* seemed to be. And so I've been thinking about it and of course I have always written extremely affectionate letters but my darling I've always written quickly, spontaneously and as I felt. And I still feel the same. I still want to sit down and dash off pages of my doings and doubts and my loving you and missing you. But each time I've started to write to you since you left this time, instead I've sat with the pen in my hand thinking over everything that happened and that we both said during your leave, and wondering exactly what made it go so abominably wrong this time. You see I've never even *heard* of any two people situated as we are. Right from the start, apart from falling in love, we've never behaved as any other people would have done in the same circumstances. We were entangled in financial complications together within the first week of knowing each other and we've been either singly or jointly getting out ever since. For four years I've had my mother living with us. She is one of the better mother-in-laws I grant you, but still it is not the same as having a 'go' alone. We've been separated a great deal, one long year at a time. Not an existence conducive to getting a cosy settled idea of each other. And apart from those lovely months at Halfway Cottage we've never had a home together that we could enjoy. You have a large family who you dearly love and rightly so. Naturally you want to see as much of them all as both you and they would wish. More tricky for it is not easy to get *anywhere* these days and I know how often you've taken a long drive to see one or all of us and then one or all of us have the bad grace to be gritty. When I've done this I hate myself more than I could ever tell you, but it is done and then you say something that maybe you didn't mean and then I do it back and then the war is on. But in short it really is the war and nothing else, unless it could possibly be that in any case we'd be going through a bit of a marriage crisis, they must occur no matter how in love one is. But this solution I've dismissed because we have never had a chance to get going yet and certainly no chance of getting into a rut. No, it is the war and the general rush of goodbyes and hallos and all the misery of separation and uncertainty.

I've really wanted to write a good and intelligent letter about us my darling, but I've failed I know. However it has done me good to write it and I feel better. What a miserable goodbye we had though my darling. I felt you were so far away from me and you didn't even seem to want to talk to me when I came to the 400.[1]

I'm sorry if I hurt you at all and I'm sorry if I made you feel I don't love you, because I do. It's true that physically we seemed a little out of line sometimes, but that too is heaven when all is well with us. And I'm quite sure that my mad desire to have another baby has a lot to do with it. I *can't* stop myself thinking 'this time perhaps' which is madness I know but I can't help it.

But darling there is no doubt in my mind at all and I've thought it over very carefully since you left, that we can and will both be wonderfully happy when once we settle together somewhere. I love you I love you I love you and I know just how dearly you've paid for this war my darling and seldom oh how seldom have you ever spoken of the utter misery and doubt and worry and discomfort most of the time you've been suffering. Six lovely years you've given, and so graciously my love. I love and respect you for all you've done and I've understood deep down in my heart the bad patches although I probably did cut up a bit rough at the time my darling. Soon soon now it will all be over and we can start to make each other happy again. In the meantime I'm here, I love you and I always will forever and ever and always and always. Your own Margaret.

1. The 400 was a London club.

Margaret to Tam — Two Gates, 4 February 1945

Tamèd my darling,

I wrote you a very long and I fear very dull letter after you went back then sat back to wait to hear what you had to say. Of course you were smart, you did the right thing. A very short not terribly affectionate letter arrived from you yesterday ignoring the whole thing.[1] I suppose you are right to ignore it, for how can we talk these things out in letters, particularly when one now and then gets lost.

But in some strange way our rows and differences during your leave stuck with me and upset me and I could not just forget, in spite of loving you so much and the two or three lovely days and evenings we had together.

It's so strange that I spend all my time longing for you when you are away, and then when you do come, the *least* thing makes one blow up or be miserable. Oh well. It will all soon be over and we can settle down to a reasonable life together my darling and forget all this.

Goodnight, God bless you again my love, I adore you,
Always,
Your M.

1. It is likely in fact that their letters crossed and Tam had not yet received Margaret's letter of 30 January. By his next letter of 5 February he had received it.

Tam to Margaret — Brussels, 5 February 1945

My Darling,

Your letter arrived last night. I'd been waiting for it and wondering what it would say. Thank you for it, it was a good letter and clearly written. If my answer is not so well written or put so clearly, you must forgive me. First of all I must answer it as if it were the absolute and certain truth. I think it is, but I don't know it is. I'm not suggesting that you did anything so silly as to deliberately lie to me, but wanting to put my mind at rest may have led to more or less than the real and absolute truth.

For a long time now, off and on, not all the time, I've had attacks of those two most horrible emotions, envy and jealousy, both quite new and strange to me, not part of me ever. I'm envious of the people who have not let the War hinder their own personal advancement and gain, and have remained near to what they love and value, and I've been jealous of you. Part of me accepts your word that you've been faithful, part of me rejects it and is certain that you have not. No part of me would really blame you, it's the doubt that troubles. I have too much of the idealist and the sentimentalist in me and not enough of the philosopher. It's hard, very hard to feel not really a soldier, no longer an actor, but a celibate husband with children growing up a long way away, someone who could be well off and give you a real and attractive home, and is in fact flat broke. Sometimes I'm quite sure my choice was right, and sometimes I'm very unsure. We should, you and I, if life were normal and not mad, have reached the lovely blissful fulfillment part of marriage. No longer the rough tempestuousness of the early stages. Those early stages when hearts are hurt so easily and words misunderstood and moods mistaken – the miseries and the anguish and the soaring ecstasies. We touched the bliss during the precious months before and after Hugo, but now (I'm speaking only for myself) I'm back again where I was, a man in love and very jealous, not a husband in love with his wife even, but a man in love with a woman.

Hugo makes no sense some days, for I can't feel on these God damn bloody little 'Leaves' that I'm anything so permanent as his father and your husband. I feel transient. All I want is to be your lover and for it all to be as full of glory and delight as it was in the beginning. And it isn't, and I wonder at the reasons, the explanations which are very many. Do you no longer want me as a lover but as an instrument to give you children? This is what I want you to answer. If so I'll try to find the reason. Has love grown cold, is seven days not long enough to establish our old relationship? Have you someone else who satisfies you sexually while I am necessary only as a companion or a father to your next baby? These are the things I wonder, and so I drink as much as I can because of the disappointment and curse myself for a fool that I haven't put our life together above all else; guarded it and secured it and sheltered it in surroundings it deserves instead of rushing off to the wars in a flurry of ineffectual heroics and rubbishy sentiments. Honour, conscience, the call of duty, call it what you like. If I'd been a hell of a good soldier it would have made so much more sense, but who knows that I wouldn't have served better by remaining an actor? I'm damned if I do. All I know is that this is the unpleasant way, and the unpleasant way is usually the right way. All these things I think and so I drink and you keep pace with me, and then a sharp tongue protects the hurt heart and the fat's in the fire and a few more hours have gone by and good-byes are getting nearer. That's about it my Darling. It's as you say, it's the war, the bloody war, the long war, and the fact that I'm just a bit of a fool. And I'm so in love with you that the foolishness surmounts the wit and intelligence.

We've had the best, let us not put up with anything else. I would, I believe I would, sooner call it a day. I don't think I could endure the agony and ignominy of a decaying passion, your decaying passion. Maybe your desire has already spent itself as far as I'm concerned and nothing I can do will make it come back. I don't know. I hope not. Maybe as you told me the other day, your whole sex life is dormant. Maybe you've had a lover whom I must make you forget. These are the questions I want the answer to.

I seem to have laid great stress on the sexual side of our life, but, and I know this so well and so truly, sex is the corner stone upon which all the other things are built. The blissful and happy life can only be reached THROUGH the ecstacy of passion. No one expects the ecstatic times to last, life would be unbearable if they did, but they are essential beginnings. There would be no golden autumns unless the glory of the spring came first. The sap in the trees rises and step by step, without haste, nature proceeds until the leaf on the tree is gold and then the winds of winter blow it away into oblivion. If I can bring you back to April days we shall live happy ever after. My fear is that the frost caught you my love. All this is high falutin and I must get on and finish, but there are odds and ends still to say.

It's a very violent change to come home having lived with men only, to a papier mâché boot box full of women. My system can't really take it. Privacy is so precious and there is none. Dressing is like trying to change your clothes with your dressing room full of friends after a first night. I can't help it and I can't bear it. I think not only my manners but my manner being attuned to male society does not readjust to the sociey of women in seven days, and so I'm a little awkward and irritable. I feel there is not enough tenderness in me to deal with them. And I feel the race against the clock, that I'm losing the race against the clock in trying to get you back to normal. I don't think I've ever enjoyed any leave after the first evening, for the next morning I begin to dread the goodbyes and once more the separation.

Don't distress yourself because you hurt me. I know very little about women, but I only know they hurt you when they love you. It's when they're kind that you know you've had it.

Write to me when you've read this, answering it, and then please write to me spontaneously and swiftly with hurried writing and bad spelling. Goodnight my darling, I want so badly to give you a happy life and a lovely home and some more remarkable babies, and to make up for the years of discomfort and lack of money, of kitchen sinks and things hanging in the bathroom, and rotten gin in dirty glasses, and catching trains and booking hotel rooms and getting taxis, and making both ends meet so hard that we ourselves have hardly met at all. But first I must see the look of April in your eyes again, then it shall be always and always, my best beloved always and forever,

Tam

Margaret to Tam Two Gates, 9 February 1945

Darling,

Your long letter arrived on Wednesday and I've re-read it many times and given it a lot of thought. A lot. Strange how much more clearly I can think when I'm alone in the house with just Hugo asleep upstairs. The mere fact of other people in the house tends to muddle my brain just now. I wonder are you like this too? Now darling you said at the beginning of your letter that you *thought* I'd written the truth but you did not *know*. I wrote the truth as I felt it then and I'm sure if I had to write the same letter to you again, that although it may read quite differently, the essential facts would stand out and remain the same. Whatever is going on now between us I honestly don't pretend to understand. I'm either 'not quite right', very stupid, or something deep down inside me warns me not to go too deeply into it, to let it just slide past if possible. The latter is right I think. Too much writing on too many pages of paper can do a lot of harm with no touch of a hand, expression on a face, or intonation of voice to guide the listener.

You speak of envy and jealousy. It would be much more extraordinary if you did *not* feel them sometimes. I too have felt the same, but only about a very small handful of people and for only a short time, for if you talk to them you feel better at once. They really envy you and yes even me because as you say it is the hard way but my God it is the right way darling. You've given me the right to hold my head high (and the rest of your family). The actual money these people have earned is the only thing you can really envy. For poor things they are going through a small hell every day trying to convince themselves that they are doing the best they can to win the war and knowing in their heart of hearts that they are not. Consequently their women suffer.

As to your place in the theatre darling, the war is nearly over and it does not even look like being taken. There is no one like yourself in the London theatre. Don't forget it took you nearly twenty years to get your position, it can't just go in the five years, particularly of wartime theatre. We've talked of your joining up being the right thing or not so many times. Perhaps you might have waited a little longer at the start, I don't know, and if I thought it were going to last much longer I'd say come out now if you can. But I do really think it will all be over soon. Then darling we'll go and make our April again for each other.

And now my darling about babies. You can try to tell me that they are the reward of love and hours well spent. I grant you they are a reward, God knows I worship Hugo. But, repeat but, I have good reason to believe that the conception of a baby is not necessarily the result of hours well spent. I love you, you love me, we both love Hugo and I hope he'll love us. But he should have a brother or a sister and I'm unable to understand why God has not seen fit to give us our wish, if not for our sakes then for his. I am miserable that we have not brought it off and nothing you can say will alter this. It is not as if we have not had many lovely nights together when it could have happened. When there has been as much love, friendship, passion and affection between us to have made a heavenly baby. However I'm miles better since you went back this time about this. I just relaxed and said to myself we are not meant to have a baby yet and that is that. You also asked me to tell you if I still want you as a lover or only as the father of my children. *Only* is surely the wrong word my darling. For how many women have you beised who you'd have died rather than have give you a son? Surely there would truly be something wrong with our marriage if at this, our eighth year together, I still wanted you as a lover only. I admit that perhaps once or twice I was not as warm a lover as I might have been, but the first night at the Grosvenor was heavenly. But Tam, during seven days' leave any rows that we have are truly ghastly for they can't be made up passionately, there is too much in one's mind and heart to take harsh words and cruelness [*sic*] lightly and make up in love with days ahead to get the harsh words washed away. I admit I drank too much, but it's only to give the illusion of a long leave, to make believe it would be much longer. Instead of which, of course, the demon alcohol makes time fly – surely the reason for the larger consumption of alcohol during war time.

I'm on my eighth page and I wonder my darling if I've answered your letter at all. I've sent of a couple of short dull letters since my long one, but I've really only been waiting for yours, which I knew would come. Thank you for it darling and for the obvious thought and care you took. If only we both get half of what we want for each other we should be ecstatically happy. And we will. You'll see my love.

How were the cakes by the way? Did they go down well? Don't not come home again if you get half a chance before the end darling. We really will be selfish and go off alone and not say a word to any of the rest of the family. Not even Hugo maybe.

If I've failed to answer your letter darling it is not unwillingness but just lack of ability. God bless and keep you always my darling, always and always, your own M.

Tam to Margaret Brussels, 11 February 1945

My Darling,

Your second letter arrived last night. You hadn't yet received my long letter and thought I was deliberately not going into the reasons why the leave was such a hideous failure. No my love I've thought about it a great deal and by this time you'll have got my letter.

I'm having my slackest period ever and the boredom is overwhelming. Two of the Patrol go on Leave this week thank goodness, for they too are feeling the strain. The initial excitement of the Russian drive has worn off,[1] leaving the usual and inevitable hangover of doubt. Not really. For it must end and within a very few months, surely to God it must. I'm making inquiries about buying a barge, to leave here of course until it's all over and then bring home and convert into a comfortable affair with an engine and things. I'm sure it would be fun and we could have loverly [*sic*] idling holidays. The children would fall in I suppose, but so should we and it wouldn't really matter. Feeling this was getting very boring I re-read your letter. Oh Dear Oh Dear. Far away, you said I seemed. The whole Leave was rather theatrically symbolised by those enormously expensive little flowers which weren't very pretty and had no scent and were dropped in the street. I wonder if you understood my letter and if you agree or disagree with most of it and if it made quite clear that I love you very much.

Goodnight my Darling,
I love and adore you and I want you so much,
Tam

1. On 31 January Russian troops crossed the River Oder north of Frankfurt, just forty miles from Berlin. Two days later they took the town of Stettin. There followed a nine days' pause before they continued to breach German defences along the Oder.

Tam to Margaret Brussels, 16 February 1945

My Darling,

Your letter answering mine arrived yesterday. I agree with you, it is very probably stupid to continue what should be a conversation by correspondance [*sic*], but when I'm not thinking of the Russians I seem to be thinking of you. There seem to be things I must have expressed badly and you seem to have missed the point. First of all my jealousy and envy are not really professional at all. What has happened to you and me during these twenty months is a very great deal more important than what has happenend to me in the six years I've been out of the theatre. I can put it better perhaps like this. I have no real fears of my future in the theatre, whereas I have genuine fears that something of your feelings, not mine, have changed and I wonder and I wonder not very confidently if I can see the successful methods of dealing with a situation, which believe it or not, I've been lucky enough never to have experienced before. For, and here it is in a nutshell, I don't think you're any longer in love with me.

Maybe I'm wrong. Maybe I'm war-weary and having nothing better to occupy my mind, I'm thinking too much and am habitually bored and depressed, but there it is and I believe it. That is what I meant about your baby. You love me and you like me and you want another child. I feel I am the means to that end rather than someone you have been physically in desperate need of as I have been of you. But for Harm's Sake get it out of your head that God is punishing you for past abortions.[1] God is forgiving and understanding and loving, though nowadays one can't quite understand as easily as one would wish.

The main part of my letter you don't answer at all. Perhaps you have decided that a letter is not the medium in which to answer. But your deliberate disregarding of it has naturally not made my feelings any less, that sometime during these twenty months you've either fallen a little in love with someone else, or had an affair for fun, or at any rate not been faithful. I told you I couldn't blame you, and I told you it was the doubt that troubled most – the doubt and the unsureness. Again forgive me if I'm wrong, and again it must be that I'm tired and weary and the Goddam war has gone on too long.

I don't believe you're in love with me any more and I don't believe you've been faithful. I can't help it and believe me I don't like it, for I'm more in love with you and feel less as if you belong to me than I have been all the other seven years we've been together.

If this letter makes you sad or worries you, I'm sorry. You must forgive me and try and understand that mountains can be made of molehills when the heart is sad and the mind is unbelievably idle. I had not meant to say as much, but it is better that I have.
Goodnight my darling, and my love to you always,
Tam

P.S. This shall be the last of these. I shall wait impatiently first for Russia and then for you.

1. Margaret alludes to this in her letter of 9 February 1945: 'I have good reason to believe that the conception of a baby is not necessarily the result of hours well spent.' More details are not available.

Margaret to Tam — Two Gates, 19 February 1945

Oh my darling,

What a day! Joyce, Mummy and me all in a high state of excitement cooking for Hugo's party tomorrow.[1] I've just made his birthday cake, now Mummy is making one and then she and I are off to a movie in Windsor. Oh darling darling Tamèd how I wish you could be here to watch him and enjoy him at his party. He and Joyce are doing some gardening. He looks such a busy serious little man. I'm in the sitting room with the door open and can see him from here.

Wonderful news still and today it looks as if it will be even better soon. Surely the whole big attack from both the Russians and ourselves will end it. I'm even more optimistic than June at the moment. They *can't* stand much more retreating and deprivation as well as the bombing surely. Oh darling imagine by next Christmas we might be Mr and Mrs again in our own home and certain of seeing each other every night and working or playing or even holidaying together. And able to make plans for tomorrow, next week or even next year. What a lovely future my darling and I can begin to see it now for the first time *truly*.

Must end now as I want to get the tea and make some jellies for tomorrow before I take my Mum to the movies.

Sending you a parcel this week darling, chocs and coffee and a few odds and ends. Let me know if there is aught you want.
God bless and take care of you my darling,
Always and always, your M.

1. Hugo was 3 on 20 February 1945.

Tam to Margaret — Brussels, 19 February 1945

My Darling,

My last letter to you was a miserable affair I'm afraid, burn it and forget it. Having nothing to do is bad at the moment and I get days of black despair about you.

You and the thought of you, and the longing, and the hope of the happiness with you after it's all over, have made the War endurable. The thought of that happiness in any kind of danger fills me with a wild kind of terror. 'Shall we not have the ebb and the flow?' I love you very much and I'm sorry I wrote you a letter which would have been much better never written. Forgive it please and forgive me.

An ugly rumour that we shall soon be out of our billets and into the fields in tents. The sun shone warmly three days ago and the dear clever high ups concluded that winter was over.
God bless you my Darling, and for always I'll go on loving you,
Always,
Tam

Margaret to Tam Two Gates, 21 February 1945

Darling One,

I wanted to write to you last night and tell you all about the birthday but I was exhausted and could only have written you a dull babble. I'd been up since 7 o'clock and into Windsor to pick up the last minute buns etc and then bending over small people from 3.30 until six and cooking until ten o'clock the night before, I had such a back ache I could hardly speak. However my darling I think the party was a success.

I made his birthday cake and iced it myself. It was sponge layers of pink, chocolate and yellow, with white icing and Happy Birthday Hugo written on the top. Written in coloured 'Hundreds and Thousands' which I put on *one at a time* with my eyebrow tweezers. Then three tiny candles, one blue, one red, one yellow. A labour of love. The table was groaning with food, eighteen children sat down to tea and about fifteen grown ups stood around and had tea too. As it was a lovely day they all had a run in the garden and then the magician. All the children adored him except – oh dear, except our chap, who burst into tears and would have none of it. Had to be taken out. He came back a little later and sat with me on the floor absolutely entranced by the tricks. Just what upset him I don't know. Your wine arrived at lunch time and Hugo's little face lit up with a wonderful smile and he said 'All the way from France, Daddy sent that.' The house is so FULL of toys we'll have to get another house if only for Hugo's toys. He's a very lucky little boy and I think we are lucky to have him too, don't you my love? Next May we'll be together again I think darling, and God willing we'll *stay* together and then we'll start another. Just four years later than Hugo. I honestly think May will see the end my love, don't you?

I know you were thinking of us my love and wondering how it went. The evening after one's son's party is a lonely time without his father to have a drink with and talk it over. I missed you *badly* last night my love, *badly*.

Good night my beloved, take care of yourself and write to me as often as you can. God bless you and keep you, I love you always and always, your own, M.

Margaret to Tam Two Gates, 22 February 1945

Beloved,

Only a short letter today, have not much news. Very broke with all the Feb financial fuck up. Telephone, electricity, rent etc, bank pretty touchy. I'm selling a lot of clothes I don't want and trying like mad to get a job.

About the barge, my feelings are mixed. At the moment I only want a home and can think no further ahead. Would it cost a lot to have it done over? But made cosy it really would be a lovely way to have a holiday. Just hire an excellent cook at each place and take a 'person' to look after us on the move.

Another lovely sunny day here so I'll take Hugo for a walk as soon as he wakes up.

The bombing of Germany must be fantastic at the moment. I could hardly sleep last night there were so many going over and coming back. Very low too they sounded. Oh surely they can't stand out much longer. Or are they going to drag it on for another year and build up the martyr stuff to the Nazis.

Hugo is awake so I must go and dress him and take him out and post this. God bless you my most beloved,
Always and always, your own M.

Tam to Margaret 23 February 1945

My Darling,

This is going to be an entirely selfish letter. Less like a letter than an administration instruction. But I'm getting very concerned about my post-war wardrobe. I have a feeling I may be swallowed up in Korda's *War and Peace* or some other lengthy costume production, in which case the studio won't help and I'm so weary of being dirty and dung coloured and drab. Half the joy of liberation will vanish if I find myself a shabby, down at heel civilian.

Somehow you will have to get coupons. I've given mine away for five years now. You must beg, borrow, steal and enter deeply into the Black Market. I shall get some on demobilisation and might repay a few. Then will you walk round to Bond St to Hammells' opposite Aspreys and order me three white Viyella shirts, if there's no Viyella, very very thin flannel. Next time you're in Charles Street pop into Lobb and charm that little man into promising my shoes for May. How you will get coupons I don't know my love, but watch Vi and see how it's done. For apart from these I want pyjamas – or do I? And a dressing gown of such great elegance that Hugo will think I've suddenly become a King. Sorry to fag you my love – I'll buy you a string of pearls one day.

Goodnight my best beloved, what part of my love you have no need of, give to my son,
Always my Darling,
Tam

Margaret to Tam Two Gates, 25 February 1945

Well my love my darling,

Cologne is getting a battering and it looks as if it will fall before the end of the week. I always imagine the news is better than we read these days. Or perhaps it is only that it is moving so rapidly these days that by the time the papers are printed we are far beyond the news.

I'm broadcasting next Sunday, March 3rd actually my darling. Poor old darling you do sound low and depressed at the moment. Well I'm feeling the Dorney Dulls at bit too my sweet, but it won't be long now, I honestly believe it this time too so let us keep our eyes glued to the top of the mountain and the lovely valley of peace and freedom on the other side. Hark at me I sound more like a letter in a cheap magazine.

It's gloriously warm here but I don't trust it. I feel sure March is going to turn on me personally and blow and sleet and freeze me back into my winter shell, along with all the other green buds and leaves that have made the same mistake as me. But honestly you'd think that some of these old old trees and flowers and bushes that have lived in England for so many hundreds of years would have learned their lesson by now, wouldn't you? I'll write again tomorrow my love and maybe I'll have a letter from you by then. I usually get one on Monday or Tuesday.
God bless you my precious one, always and always,
Your own M.

Tam to Margaret 25 February 1945

Margaret my Darling,

Two letters from you last evening. The one about Hugo's party was really good and made me see the whole thing from the anxious preparations to the exhausted sleepy head flopped on the pillow, while you, my love, felt the anti-climax and needed to be taken out to a cosy dinner and told what a magnificent success the whole thing had been.

Lordamercy was there ever in all the world anything so deeply magnificent and superabundant as a mother's love. Make the most of it Darling, indulge it to the utmost for in another five years he'll be allergic to affection and your place in his heart will be temporarily taken by some other odious little brat whose possession of a catapult or a white rat places him upon a pedestal, which if you're wise you'll properly recognise, and in ten years he'll be criticising your hats and in fifteen my port. Then a little later, if we've been good and amusing and intelligent parents and after he has viewed the world through his own eyes and not through the eyes of a thousand other schoolboys whom for a dozen years he's been trying to emulate, when individuality triumphs over convention, then he'll come back and we shall have bound him to us for the rest of our lives and all the anxieties and the disappointments and the snubs will have been worthwhile.

You ask me to tell you of the contest. Well obviously I can't tell you anything about this end and I know no more than you of the Russians. But I feel fairly sure that May or perhaps June will see the end of it, with perhaps isolated pockets of lunatics clinging frantically to strong points in the Bavarian Alps. Don't sell too many of your clothes my Darling and please not the plum coloured one you wore the night you started making love to me, not that one please.

Goodnight beloved, take care of yourself. Write soon and often,

Always,

Tam

Margaret to Tam — Two Gates, 26 February 1945

Tamèd my Darling,

It is so hard to time letters exactly these days to arrive on a certain day, but this one is meant to be opened on your birthday my love. Happy Birthday Beloved and may it be your last one spent away from us. From now on each March 6th you'll waken in bed beside me and I'll grab you and kiss you and give you a lovely present and wish you a happy birthday and Hugo will dart in and do the same thing. And we'll have a party and a gloriously gay and happy day and night together always in the future darling. Your present this year is not terrific darling, but if you don't like it you can hang it in the lavatory when we get our home. A girl called Elizabeth Tapley has painted me for you. It's very like me I think in a flattering way (unlike Nora's). Three quarter face no hat in the dress I married you in. It is ¾ length sitting hands loosely clasped in my lap. She is having a photograph taken of it for me to send to you my darling, but you know what ages they take these days so I'm afraid they won't reach you for the day and I can't imagine for a moment you'd like me to send you the picture itself darling. Happy birthday to you darling in the meantime and all my love. How I wish you'd been at home and I could hang it up and let you find it for yourself.

Your letter dated 23rd arrived this morning. I shall carry out your instructions for your post-war wardrobe to the best of my ability darling, and *love* doing it. But first of all I must start a coupon campaign. You too might scrounge a few, just 2 or 3 here and there to help. Johnny has a lot I think, try him. Happy Birthday again my darling and I hope you'll like your pressy when you see it.
All my love always and always, your M.

Tam to Margaret — Belgium, 3 March 1945

Darling Margaret,

It's been a good week, this. Quite like the old Normandy days and it's been a God send to have some interest and excitement again. That, and the debate on Yalta,[1] upon which my feelings are a little mixed. There is no doubt the Polish Government have been a nuisance, there is no doubt Churchill and Roosevelt did the only practical thing which was to say 'Yes Joe' (and thank God they did) and there's no doubt Poland has been shopped. But Europe must heal and cannot be allowed to bleed to death for the sake of a pennyworth of English Honour. Better to be honest than honourable, but I can take it better if the honesty isn't faked up in Churchillian eloquence to sound like honour – the whole thing begins to stink. Eden[2], you notice, stuck to figures and facts, while Churchill offered excuses and justifications. I'm beginning to think Eden is strengthening and may be the solution. But I find it a little appalling to see the causes of the next war appearing before the conclusion of this one, whilst at the same time I see that it is the only possible and practical answer at the moment. Power politics – you can't ever get away from them, so you have to get round them. I dare say the reason the Prime Minister smokes so many cigars is to take away the nasty taste in his mouth.

No coupons available here – we only get them when serving in England. I'll write to Mother and the girls to see what they can do. If I threaten to attend her Speech Day in a dinner jacket Loo will contrive and contribute.

I've been waiting for an answer to a letter I wrote to you on February 16th, but you've apparently decided not to. In it I wrote that I was quite sure you were no longer in love with me – this you practically told me when I was on leave. I wondered why. Have you been unfaithful and got involved in an affair, were you in love with anyone else or was it just the separation? And so I wrote a long letter to you, but in you reply you avoided the issue, so I wrote again and this time you ignore the whole letter. Perhaps you think a letter is a dangerous method of making such a confession and that when I return you'll be able to persuade me that I was either mistaken or that your affair was unimportant – a phase – a boob – the war – and we should forgive and forget and go out to dinner. Very likely. But what I shall never forget are these months you've been keeping me in doubt and uncertainty – and I shall never forgive you for being such a bloody fool and such a mean little bitch and not writing and telling me what it's all about. It's quite probable I shan't get back until the Autumn. In the meantime if I am to be kept in this uncertainty subconsciously my mind will inevitably make re-adjustments. When the re-adjustments are complete then I see little chance of our relationship ever being what it used to be. What, six weeks ago when I came back, was a jealous doubt, through your ignoring the issue and questions in my letters, has become now almost a certainty in my own mind. So do please answer this, my third attempt.

God bless you and my love to you all,
Tam

1. Churchill, Roosevelt and Stalin met at Yalta to determine their spheres of influence in post-war Europe.
2. Anthony Eden (1897–1977), Foreign Secretary in wartime coalition government.

Tam to Margaret Advancing through France, 8 March 1945

My Darling,

By the time you get this we shall be out in the wet fields and soon I suppose we shall find ourselves back on biscuits and Bully and the mail will go haywire and there'll be a shortage of cigarettes and underclothes and we'll get dirtier and smellier – all the usual shambles of a swift advance. The Fruits of Victory are really very sour. However, maybe a little Rhine wine will prove a welcome change from Pommery and there'll be a certain satisfaction in being in Germany. One has travelled a somewhat circuitous route to get there but I imagine, for I really have forgotten now it's so long ago, that one did have a Reich in mind as an ultimate destination. Anyway the Goddam End is very near. The Rhine will be tricky and may take time but after that, like the water jump at Aintree, it's a straight run home. Then Heigh Ho! for the Brave New World. We shall have to be very brave I fancy, for it promises to be quite intolerable. I never pick up a paper without seeing some encouraging little headlines like High Taxation to Remain for Years, Whisky Shortage in 1948, Will there be Domestic Servants after the War, No Private Cars for Two Years, Post-War Housing Problems, Government will Restrict Travel. If we are to be happy My Love, we must make our own enchantment.

Goodnight My Darling, be good, and take care of yourself. I love you so much. I hope you've answered my last letter. God Bless, Always and always,
Tam

Tam to Margaret Germany, 13 March 1945

My Darling,

In my last letter I painted an unhappy picture of damp tents in sodden fields. Thank God I was wrong and we are once again in billets, the inhabitants having being given six hours to quit, which I'm rather glad I didn't witness. I daresay during the Blitz of 1940 it might have been gratifying to see a few German towns laid flat in dusty rubble, but nowadays they merely fill one with dejection like all the others one has seen. Horror has reached a new high – 5000 tons on Dortmund yesterday.[1] It's ungraspable, thank God. The mind and imagination are mercifully limited and cannot comprehend such appalling concentrated human agonies.

It's strange how the flags which began in Tunis and continued to greet our arrival through Italy, Normandy, France, Belgium and Holland, should still appear in the Fatherland. This time they're white though, fluttering from church spires and farms and cottage windows they slightly turn the stomach. The people look well fed and healthy and quite prosperous and there is an abundance of fowls, ducks and geese – eggs for tea – though no cattle, not even dead in the fields as they were in Normandy. In this village nearly every house had a supply of coal, which I must say rather infuriated me, but of course had obvious advantages.

I love you my Darling Heart and I promise you a life led lovingly and happily and busily and kindly. I worship you and always will, Tam

1. On 11 March one thousand bombers took part in the biggest ever daylight raid on a German city.

Tam to Margaret — Germany, 19 March 1945

My Darling,

A letter written on huge paper from you last night and one from Prudie too, whom I now hear from on the average twice a week. She writes in prep, I rather fancy.

Any luck with coupons? Getting another officer shortly which will be a help if things busy up. Lunched with Michael Astor today who's hoping to be adopted as Conservative Candidate for Tonbridge Wells! The atmosphere is very tense and full of excitement. I believe it will be over very soon now, to all intents and purposes. How long the United Nations will take to decide a date for A Day (as it is now being called) is another matter.

You ask me to write you a long loving letter and I reply with this short, dull and ill-phrased thing which might have been written to an Aunt or a Bank Manager. If you want to know what I think of the last thing before I fall asleep (which is very bad for me) and the first thing in the morning and a great part of each day, it's you my Beloved. If you want to know why I long for the War to end and to get out of the Army, it's to be with you my Darling. If you want to know upon what all my plans and hopes and ambitions are focused, it's you my Margaret. If you want to know what I've missed these last years, it's not my work or my comfort or my income or my pleasant food or well made clothes or my friends, but you my Angel. If you want to know whom I love more than life, whom I'd sooner sleep with than anyone in the world and

whom I'd sooner look at and talk to and take out to dinner than anyone else it's you my Sweet. But I suspect you already know all that and I've been taught in the Army never to duplicate information. So goodnight and if you behave and are kind and sweet and very loving and look after me and get me my coupons and order my clothes and find a nice house for us I shall go on feeling as I do now for Always and Always.
Tam

Tam to Margaret Germany, 23 March 1945

My Darling,

I saw Cologne the other day, which needs seeing to believe and filled me with the most profound and utter misery. I've seen many villages and small towns reduced to dusty rubble but nothing on the scale of Cologne which was once the home of a million people. I saw nothing that looked habitable, nothing. The Cathedral is, I suppose, remarkably untouched and is repairable – but how God knows – and I'm quite sure only God does know for no precision bombing could have spared it – all around it is destroyed and desolate and the silence is awful – by that I mean I really was filled with awe – and very nearly with terror. For to see destruction on such a scale, such magnitude *is* terrifying for it illustrates the hideous, gigantic power of the machine and man's inability to control it. Pure Frankenstein. A shell landed with a bang a few streets away as I was looking up at the Cathedral, frightening the pigeons who circled round for a bit and then resettled on the spires, and it really seemed that they were superior creatures to mankind – for they neither destroyed as we do, nor were they liable to destruction. The thing has gone too far and it is sickening and horrible and Godless. Pray God it ends soon which I think it will, very soon – which reminds me, have you done anything about my tailors and haberdashers? Nearly a month since I wrote about it.

I saw Hugh Stewart. He's head of the Second Army Film Unit and is also contracted by Korda as Associate Producer. He told me the Studio at Elstree will not be ready for Production for at least a year and Alex therefore will only be able to make one picture at a time on floor space he has at Denham. Now supposing he starts a lengthy production in June with nothing in it for me, he's not going to employ any great pressure to get me out, it means I must get a play or picture elsewhere. I shall tell Connie in my letter to start *now* for by June or the end of May or perhaps next week it will be over and I'm damned if I spend six months, six valuable months, drawing 5/- a day Intelligence Pay in the Fatherland.

No letters from anybody. You seem to write two a week both posted at the same time, haven't heard from Mum for a couple of weeks and Gwynne not for ages. The only person who writes regularly is Prue who is new to it and not bored to tears with years of letter writing.

No more now darling, my love always and always,
Tam

P.S. Reckon in your mind the war will be over in a month and I shall be back in England in ten weeks and shall want a nice house to live in and beautiful clothes to wear and a very good part in a not too stinking play and that you're the only person who can help me.

Tam to Margaret Germany, 27 March 1945

My Darling,

First letter from you tonight in over a week, as usual written on 21st and posted 24th, or, as I strongly suspect, both written on 24th and ante-dated. I find it quite maddening. I know the mail is working perfectly so there's absolutely no excuse for the miserable littleness I'm getting. This you can tell the rest of the family except Prue, I've had more letters in the last month from her than from the rest of you put together. And from you personally I heard oftener and received them more quickly when I was in North Africa than nowadays. This is a thoroughly well earned and I hope well aimed rocket. From now on I write in answer only. Well, that had to be said and that's that.

The battle goes well, saw the Air Display, very thrilling though so precise and punctual it was rather like the tattoo. I think it'll be over in a month easily. Have written to Connie so get on to her at once. I've had another idea. I'd rather like to go to India or Burma with E.N.S.A. – and you, if you're pleasant and nice – for three or four months, if there's anything going and if it's going in May. What do you feel? I dread the aftermath of the campaign. I had it in Africa and Italy and I can't take it again. And it would be fun and it would be travel and it would be good for you to ease the claustrophobia of the last five years and it might be wise to practise a little in Cairo or Delhi or Mandalay rather than Shaftesbury Avenue. And it might be a good transition from Army and separation back to the grind of the Brave New World. Tell Connie to cable Alexander Korda if there's any chance. If she can find me a picture or play in May, well and good, or if you hate the idea then forget it. But I'm sure it will be over in the next month and I want ACTION.

God Bless, love to Hugo and you, you idle bitch,
For Always Always,
Tam

Margaret to Tam Two Gates, 27 March 1945

Oh my darling,

I've not written to you for three days now, three of the longest I've ever spent because I've been out of my mind with worry. I did not want to tell you because I know what torture it is to get bad news and then have to wait for the next letter for more news. But I've thought and thought and finally I knew that I either had to tell you or not write at all. And anyhow things are better now and you need not worry so much.

Hugo has been quite badly burnt on the hand by an exposed electric point. I was in London doing a broadcast and Mummy was looking after him alone, but fortunately a friend of hers was here and was able to hold him while M rang doctors taxis etc. If he'd been in the room alone I don't think he'd have been saved but M was wonderful and the moment she heard him yell grabbed him up. His little body was stiff with the shock. Mummy whisked him in to Windsor hospital, ordered a specialist, signed the permission for an anaesthetic etc and Mr Shell operated. He was only under for about twenty minutes, but a longish time for a baby. They took away all the burnt flesh (first and second fingers of the left hand) and made a skin graft from under the same arm. This was done on Sunday and if the graft is a success it will have saved Hugo a lot of pain. If not we are just where we started from. Shell says he will not remove the dressing for a week as he does not want to disturb the graft. Infection is very unlikely and we are praying it won't set up. It was a third degree burn and worse than they thought at first, but so far he has not shown any signs of shock and has had good nights and seems quite happy. Shell said he wanted to keep him in the hospital, so he is in the children's ward of King Edward the Seventh's, Windsor. They asked if we'd like him to be put in a private ward but we said not as I'm sure he'd hate to be alone. We are not allowed to see him, but of course I've seen him without him seeing me. They think it is too upsetting for children to see their mothers, so I've agreed though it breaks my heart. I go in every day and peek at him and take him goodies and he looks quite happy thank God, but Oh how I wish I knew if it will be alright at the end of the week. He was fantastically brave and did not cry even when he was taken into the operating theatre and saw all the whiteness and masks etc. Just said it hurt a bit and asked a lot of questions. And a third degree burn must hurt like hell.

Oh I'm sorry my love, I've told you now and I suppose you'll worry until you get my next letter, but I *can't tell* you how much better I feel. Very selfish of me I fear, but there it is and I'm going to seal this up and send it off before I have time to think and then go and have a drink. I'll write every day until he's quite O.K. Forgive me my darling but I could not go on each day and not tell you.

I have no news my love, I just live for news of Hugo at the moment. But he is in good condition and heals well and quickly so I'm sure all will be well in a day or two. Forgive me for burdening you, but this too my beloved is part of my love.
I adore you for always, your own M.

Tam to Hugo Germany, Good Friday, March 1944

My Darling Hugo,

What a silly fellow you are to go fooling about with electric points, let it be a lesson to you and from now on express absolute ignorance of all such contrivances and you'll find it not only saves you a lot of trouble, but there's always someone about who knows more than you do. You and I seem to be lucky with electricity. About twenty minutes before this war began I trod on a live wire on a bridge at Staines, but luckily it wasn't in the mood and I was alright otherwise you wouldn't be here now, which I should hate.

I shall be home soon for the Germans are already beaten and it won't take long now. I miss you so much and I hate to be away when you go and hurt yourself. I haven't yet said what I wrote this letter for and that is I'm sorry my Dear Boy you should have had such Damn bad luck and I hope it's better now and doesn't hurt

any more and in the meantime I shall think of something to make up for it a bit when I get back.
Love to Mummy and to you my Darling, stupid son,
Daddy.

Tam to Margaret Germany, Good Friday, March 1944

Oh My Darling,

You poor little devil, but don't worry, you should be thinking yourself, as I do, the luckiest parent on earth that he didn't kill himself. But Oh My God I share it with you, the terror he must have felt, the horribleness of being left in a strange white forbidding hospital, so much worse than anything that could have happened to oneself. The price of loving is the sharing of pain and unhappiness and the vicarious is, if anything, worse than the actual. Poor little boy. But don't worry, he's alright and he'll never remember it in five years. But it's all *Balls* about not going to see him. Bloody Nurses' Dictates to save themselves trouble. You're his most important person in the world and you must show him that you're always there, like a solid rock. It's not to spare his feelings they tell you to keep away but their own trouble. Let him sob when you leave but when he wakes in the morning he'll know you'll be there soon and his day will be happier. You must learn to dispute *all* regulations *always*. One more thing, don't *ever, ever, ever* wait three days before letting me know of catastrophes. I'm not someone to shield from worry but to share it with at once.

Very late now, had a long and hell of a day and I'm on again at five. The enemy is beaten and it's a question no longer of months or weeks but days – ten – fifteen – thirty at the outside. On the move again, into tents. I'll be with you by the end of May. Give Hugo my love and tell him to write to me and tell me what he'd like me to bring him back from Germany. Don't worry my Darling Margaret, from now on I'll be with you in the crises. How children ever grow up is as big a miracle as how they are born and one must shrug a shaking shoulder and pretend to be brave,
All my love always,
Tam

Tam to Margaret Germany, Easter Monday, 2 April 1944

My beloved,

Another letter from you last night giving me more news of Hugo. Poor little fellow and poor darling Margaret, I can tell by your letters how you've suffered. You must promise me that if ever I'm seriously ill you will insist I have my own way over everything, other than treatment. I think the medical profession and the nursing profession are the two greatest there are, but they have one abiding sin and that's love of power, and they imagine if a patient is too weak in body to wash himself he is too weak in spirit to give orders which must be obeyed. And they thoroughly enjoy the shake of the head and the non-commital answers – 'Not yet awhile' or 'We'll see what the Doctor says' or 'Now that wouldn't be good for you' and 'You must be patient'. There was an actor in Australia who was dying in a nursing home and he asked the nurse to get him a whisky and soda, which she refused, and with all his remaining strength he screamed 'If you don't get me a whisky this instant I'll bloody well haunt you for the rest of your life – beginning tomorrow morning' and he had his drink and died in the night.

Give Hugo my love, Oh Dear he's so very young to have encountered the wretchedness of a hospital and an operating theatre, poor little sod. Has he had much pain? God Bless you my Darling, take care of yourself and don't fret about him. Anxious to hear what you think of the E.N.S.A. idea, or what plans Connie is making. I might be home in eight weeks. I love you my sweet and I always always shall,

Tam

Tam to Margaret Germany, 5 April 1945

A letter and a card from you my Darling and from them I gather Hugo is alright and by now must be home with you.

Weather back to February, cold and very wet, the last kick of the bloodiest winter ever. My tent leaks like a sieve and the other morning after a night of ceaseless rain and endless shifting about, I awoke with my hair soaking, the drips on my face and my clothing drenched. The damn things have been packed up since last October and the guy ropes have rotted, however the war slips to its final conclusion, which is all that matters.

I've done and seen enough now to satisfy curiosity. Oddly it's not turning out to be as exciting as I thought, not really like France.

Perhaps I'm tired. I think perhaps I am. Anyway, tired of the food and the discomfort and the eternal male and the wireless not working and the grumblings of my Patrol who certainly show signs they are tired and bored. So give Connie no peace.

All my love my most adorable Margaret, I'll get back to you soon and in the meantime behave and write and love me for I shall worship you,
Always and my love,
Tam

Tam to Margaret Germany, 8 April 1945

Margaret My Darling,

I like the sound of the P.O.W. Picture at Ealing, you always get a good clash of characters in those kind of stories, but I've got a lot of detail of a big concentration camp, civilian, where they tortured and murdered and used the prisoners for experimental stuff. Human Guinea Pig business. And a true story about it all simply must be made, and remade every three years. I have joined the great boring majority of the Army who say 'People in England don't realise what the German race are like'. But I think this: That the People of England, stunned by the TON weight of lies and rubbish printed in the daily press, no longer believe or digest what they read. I would make this picture as horrifying as possible and half a dozen times during it I would have a voice, over the dialogue and the action, saying, 'This is a true story you're seeing, this man's name was so-and-so and this conversation you're hearing took place on Sunday April 10th 1943. Shock and offend the susceptibilities of the complacent. Let yourself be accused of merely depicting sadism for sensational reasons – who cares? People must realise that there's as much difference between us and the Germans as between an old grey mare and a roaring, man-eating lion, and if we're going to live in the same paddock, the lion must have his teeth and claws cut regularly, kept tied up and given enough to eat so it doesn't get hungry. A dull metaphor, but I'm terrified we shall forget. Already captured German Officers have said they considered Yalta a triumph for Germany, because the one thing they all feared was a partitioning of their country. That Germany will remain a united country they consider is a *sine qua* non that she will one day fight again and next time conquer the world.

A letter from Gwynne yesterday telling me Silver has sprained her ankle and will have to lie it up for three weeks. Oh Dear Oh

Dear Oh Dear! Poor Darling. Her plans all upset and she must be miserably bored and lonely. I seem to ask you to do so many things for me nowadays, but if you possibly can please go down for the night and see how she is and cheer her up.

God Bless you my Darling. *Get Me Out.* I feel like getting busy. I have much to do and I want to get into your bed again and see my children and have something nice to eat. I shall love you till I die and beyond that,
For Always,
Tam

Tam to Margaret Germany, 9 April 1945

Beloved,

Moving again tomorrow. My own personal guess, which you must know by experience is invariably quite wrong, is that I shall have completed my own part of the war within three weeks, so I am at anybody's service from May onwards.

How's our Hugo? Home and happy now I hope.

If only the Russians would have a go at the Berlin Sector[1] it'd be all over in a week or ten days. D'you see they're giving Turkey[2] the works, and want a Free Dardanelles. Time was when England would have gone to war for that, and time may prove we shall. We don't like Russia encroaching on the Near East – it's a road that leads to too many places. Certainly the most significant news of a fairly colourful week.

I liked this remark of a German Prisoner being interrogated the other day: 'In the old days you sometimes arrived at the station to find the train gone – nowadays the train's there but the station's gone.'

Darling I can hardly contain myself when I think I shall be home and with you soon. God Almighty what misery the last few years have been. The Barren Boredom of them, the separations, but I've been luckier than most, God knows, so I'm a rat to grumble. Goodnight and my love to you always, to Hugo too,
Tam

1. In fact the Russians did not sweep into Berlin until 30 April.
2. Turkey did not enter the war until 23 February 1945 when she joined the Allies, a move which entitled her to a place in the United Nations.

Margaret to Tam Two Gates, 13 April 1945

Darlingest,

Two lovely letters from you this morning, they have both set me in a *flurry* of *activity* but there is really very little I can do now. I rang Claridges this morning and had a short talk with Korda, he told me he was seeing Connie today, and I'm meeting him one day next week for a drink. I'll ring Con later this afternoon for a drink and find out how she got on. No doubt she'll write to you and tell you herself. But one thing Korda did say was *yes* I *do* want him and soon too.

Loo's birthday party last night, we went to the Crown and Cushion for the party and present opening. She had some lovely presents and I gave her a cheque for a guinea from you, not a lot I know darling, but I'm a bit broke to do much at the moment. Poor old Prue has another roaring cold, beastly luck, but otherwise is looking well. Loo is looking marvellous and very grown up, she looked very pretty last night in a red dress Mummy and I had altered for her the night before, and a blue ribbon in her hair. I'm sitting in the glorious hot sun as I write this darling and how glad I am to know you are at last having good weather too. I was truly worried about you getting so wet each night my darling. Oh golly golly golly if only Connie and Korda really do get cracking, there is no knowing how soon we may be together again, maybe only a few weeks. I do hope the patrol are in better form now, no doubt your own mood or frame of mind had carried to them without your realising it. I can understand everyone showing their boredom now, it is so near the end. I've written all this without one mention of the Roosevelt disaster.[1] Oh dear how sad he has not lived to see the end, a great man, and a *great* loss, how desolate his family must be. I wonder what the political reaction will be and I wonder how Truman will work out. Tell me what you think.

All my love always, your M.

1. On 12 April President Roosevelt died, leaving as his successor the less-experienced Harry S. Truman.

Margaret to Tam Two Gates, Friday 14 March 1945

Well my beloved,

The wheels are really in motion. I talked to Connie this afternoon and she had seen Korda and this is what I gathered from my conversation with her. Korda definitely will apply for you at once.

It is for a part (not very good I gather) in *Lottie Dundas*, with Vivien Leigh and Larry producing. Korda says he has nothing better for you at the moment but it is an opportunity of getting you out. Also I feel he wants to use you rather than let anyone else, with the thought in mind 'After all he is under contract to me.' It is, I gather, supposed to start in June. Now with any luck we can start to plan our lives. Oh the glorious heavenly wonderful thought of it.

They say Churchill is not going to Roosevelt's funeral, now I wonder why? Things must be going to crack here very soon that require him to be here. I would not be at all surprised to hear some really big news before you get this letter darling. Oh Jimminy Cricket, I think I'll just sit down and cry for joy when I know you are *definitely* coming home. Give me time to make some nice plans darling, because there will be a lot of people with very much the same ideas as ours.

I'm going to start right away looking for a decent furnished house, I thought perhaps Hampstead if I can't find one in these parts. What ideas from you darling?

I'm sure Korda will get cracking now darling and *of course* I'll keep my eye on Connie. I agree she does owe us some service for a thousand a year. I can't see how it can last more than a few days now, so darling I'll be seeing you in all the old familiar places soon, soon, soon. All my love darling always and always,
Your M.

Tam to Margaret Germany, 14 April 1945

Darling,

Months ago I wrote to ask you to instruct Connie to have Gwynne's £10 a week paid to her direct. I did this via you rather than straight to Connie as I thought you would prefer to give the instruction yourself. Twice since I've asked for confirmation that you'd done this, no answer. I hear from Gwynne that she's broke. Please let me know at once when you gave this instruction and how much money Gwynne has received since Christmas, you will also tell Connie to send Gwynne an extra £15 this week. I want an answer from you immediately telling me this has been done and answering my questions. If not I shall write direct to Connie telling her she must administer these slender amounts in future and not you, and I shall send my orders to her instead.

How is my Mother's ankle? Where is she? Have you telephoned

– written – been to see her? What do you think I should be doing for Ruby in the same circumstances and you were abroad? Maybe she's at Cardiff, recovered and quite alright, but for the love of God use what little intelligence he gave you and let me know. You were admirable about news of Hugo, for that was of interest to you and near your heart. Try and remember this, to me, is of equal if not more importance.

Sorry this is such an unpleasant letter, but I'm thoroughly out of patience. Now for God's sake answer my questions about Gwynne's finance and my Mother's whereabouts and welfare at once and post the bloody thing the same day you write it. Love Always, but certainly not at the moment, Tam

P.S. Please give Loo £1 for me for her birthday. Can't remember if I asked you to do this before. Inclined to think I forgot damn it and if I didn't I expect you did.

Margaret to Tam Two Gates, April (undated) 1944

Now look, you wrote to me as if I were your secretary who not only was not following your instructions but was also embezelling [*sic*] your money. It seems to me some years ago I foolishly undertook to try and make both ends meet in this very oddly assorted family of ours. It has, I grant you, been made easier by the fact that we are all fundamentally nice people with one aim in view, 'To get through the war and see that our children lack nothing'. This, so far, has been done!! A miracle! Not made without some human efforts however. You my husband have, I know, done the unpleasant job but with some satisfaction no doubt. There has been little satisfaction in our jobs, certainly not for show. Yes, Hugo is a fine little boy and the girls are both grand, even Prue's asthma is abating and she is a gallant, gay, charming little girl in spite of all her bloody doctors and doctors and more doctors.

I have to write this letter quickly, for it is all seething in my mind and I must get it off my chest. So forgive all mistakes and simply *forgive* when you have finished this. Either you dislike finance so much that you don't read what I write about it, or my letter re same has never reached you. Now these figures are not dead in line for it would take far too long to go into the odd shillings and pence, but there, or rather *here* they are. In Jan I paid Silver her £24 plus £28 for Loo's fees and she has had £24 a month since and now an extra £24 for Loo's fees again by May 1st. That is

£149. I had to get the first £28 for Loo's fees from Connie and consequently for the last six weeks have had only £25 a week. Gwynne has had £105 since Jan *but* Loo's fees were paid and some of Prue's. The £11 a month from you was taken two months in advance you will remember, January's having gone at Christmas. These amount to £254 or thereabouts. Since Jan I have £254 and with this I have paid, apart from bills which I will mention later, for our own needs.

House 3. 13. 6.

Joyce 2. 0. 0.

Food milk meat veg laundry etc 4. 0. 0.

Total 9. 13. 6. Say £10. 0. 0. A week this is, the bare living with nothing to spend.

Well, since Jan this amounts to about fifteen weeks, that is £150. That makes the £254 left to £104. Now here are the other things I've *had* to pay, to say nothing of the little money one must have for just pocket money.

Interest on my stuff in pop[1]	£14
Telephone account of 6 mnths	£27
Dr Tait	£5
Neil for taxis run up while you were home	£5. 14s.
Charles Scott for drink so you could take some back	£10

THESE ARE ONLY A FEW.

That leaves me with the magnificent sum of £37 for me to run riot on in 15 weeks, just over £2 a week. Now none of these figures are exact Tam, for I've had to do some fiddling to make them go round, particularly as I've still got an overdraft at the bank of £200. A lot of unpleasant interviews and promises of less cheques cashed etc. This is a brief outline of what is happening to your money and now you ask me to send Gwynne an extra £15. Where the *hell from?* I wrote you a long letter about this before, only couched in more soothing words. She gets the first cheque every month from Connie and Silver the second and me the third if I'm lucky and the bills the fourth if *they* are lucky. In fact I wrote you a letter answering all financial questions in full and hated doing it. Tonight I take some pleasure in doing so. *And* no doubt you are now thinking I'll write the bitch such a letter she won't forget in a hurry, how bloody dare she etc etc. Well you *can*, but I can do so much and no more Tam, and there it is. We are not thank God seriously in debt (and thank you and Korda) not anything like starving.

I adore lovely clothes and props as much as you do, and I love a good time as much as you do, but when I've not spent *any* money on myself except for woollies and interest on stuff in pop, I *hate* you writing me sticky letters as if I'm holding out on you all, or being a spendthrift.

As for your mother, *immediately* I heard about her ankle I wrote and suggested going down and staying with her or helping her to get away – as she will tell you – and she wrote back to thank me and say she was off to Cardiff and could manage and thanked me very much for thinking of it.

Your daughters and Gwynne are still at the Crown and Cushion but are moving to another place in Windsor on Tuesday. They all seem to be having a gay holiday and enjoying themselves. Loo and Prue come out here quite often. Mummy is well and sends her love. Hugo is full of beans and getting quite brown. I'm taking him to the hospital tomorrow to have the plaster off, am most anxious to know how his fingers will be. He has been very brave about it all. I am well and did not get the job I went to see Linnett about.

My love always,
But not at the moment, M.

Yes it is a magnificent achievement[2] and I am proud, bloody proud, of being an Australian.

P.S. I gave Loo a cheque for a guinea from you. No you did *not* ask me to.

P.P.S. I know this is a stink of a letter AND a bad one and full of holes you can pick *if* you chose.

1. Margaret had pawned some of their belongings.
2. Margaret is referring to her keeping the family afloat in difficult circumstances. Why she related it to being Australian is difficult to say.

Tam to Margaret — Germany, 17 April 1945

My Darling,

I fear my last letter was gritty, but I'm worried about Mum and Gwynne being broke and I can't seem to get any news.

I thought last Sunday's newspapers overdid it a trifle with headlines 'Any Minute Now', 'This is the Last Weekend', but even so it's very near. In fact it *is* over and this is the rather bothersome Harlequinade – Stalin still not yet announced his offensive, and Hitler issuing orders of the day – and soon the day will come and I shall get drunk like millions of others, I suppose, with my impatience mounting and my restlessness increasing with every mouthful. Lovely weather now. I'm sitting in a very pretty garden of a nice farmhouse in my shirt, an orchard of cherry is bursting blossom, and tulips and pansies, and hens cackling and a drone of bees in the fruit trees – very pleasant and peaceful, and there's hock for dinner.

You asked me about Roosevelt, but I've always said I thought he was the greatest man alive, his work was almost done, and done magnificently. Lease lend[1] was his greatest effort and the skilful jockeying of America towards war, before Pearl Harbour made it easy for him.[2] Washington and Lincoln they compare him to, but Washington fought England and Lincoln fought the South, as far as we're concerned we've never had a better friend and so for England he must remain the greatest American. Far and away the worst part of his death is Mr Truman, whom one imagines to be unqualified and ill-equipped to deal with the domestic problems on his hands. The Peace and International Policies must surely have been all tied up at Yalta.

It's a funny feeling, this waiting to begin life again; like waiting to be hatched. I wonder what Alexander Korda's idea of soon is? Mine is next month. People are being demobilised now alright without trouble and this regiment has a superfluity of Officers so it couldn't matter less.

No more my Darling, thank you for telling me about Loo and her birthday and for giving her the Guinea. They're darlings both of them.

What a perfect month April is to have a baby – next year if you get me home soon. A pram under a tree in blossom with Spring sunshine shining through the leaves.

God Bless you my Darling and my love to you always,
Tam

1. Under Lend Lease America became the 'Arsenal of Democracy', supplying arms without asking for payment. She did, however, strip Britain of her gold reserves and overseas investments. Thanks to the scheme the United Kingdom maintained the misleading appearance of being a Great Power until almost the end of the war.
2. On 7 December 1941 the Japanese attacked the American base at Pearl Harbor in the Pacific, bringing the United States into the war.

Tam to Margaret — Germany, Primrose Day[1] 1945

My Beloved,

A letter has just arrived telling me Connie has seen Alexander Korda and is applying for my release. Dear God what news! The end of term, the discharge from hospital, the King's Pardon, the Tote Double, the Abolition of the Slave Trade, Rescue from Shipwreck, Safety after Danger, food after hunger, the Resurrection of the Dead and Life Everlasting – what are these to the end of an inglorious and abysmal career in the British Liberation Army? But maybe there will be the familiar Slip Twixt the Cup of Happiness and the Expectant Lip. So I will try to say no more and think no more, which is on second thoughts quite impossible to any but a cold-blooded fish-like fellow with nought in his veins but khaki, blanco, and no more spirit than you can buy for 5/6 at the Berkeley. You'll never know, you'll never know my love and it's only now because it's springtime and the end's in sight that I begin to know. Sorrow, boredom, separation, illness – they all become bearable only through habit and only on recovery do you fully realise how beastly it's all been.

My Dear Girl – who cares if the part is poor or the script is putrid, it's the gate opening. I'd play the hind legs of a funny horse. Not a high price to pay for liberty and comfort and cleanliness, financial security and domestic bliss. Keep me informed for I'm impatient my love. 'There's a lift in the blood! – O this gracious and thirsting and aching unrest – All Life's at the bud! And my heart full of April is breaking my breast'.[1]

All my love to you both, and to you always,
Tam

1. Primrose Day was 19 April, anniversary of the death of Disraeli, whose favourite flower it was said to have been.
2. From a poem by W.E. Henley, a poet beloved of Tam's parents. It is from Poem IX in the sequence 'Hawthorn and Lavender'.

Margaret to Tam — Two Gates, 23 April 1945

Well my love,

I talked to Con yesterday as I think I told you, and asked her to place your bets. I also asked her to find out how your release application – sounds like a liniment! – was going but she has not given me any news yet.

It looks as if the war is not nearly as near the end as everyone was led to believe by the newspapers a week ago. I'm sure they will fight in every corner now until someone, God knows who, certainly no Nazi leader, says we've had enough boys. Rommel could have done it for them perhaps,[1] but who now? Surely it must be the army command who finally throws in the sponge. Fanatic bastards, they must fight on or die like dogs, hoping to be made martyrs I suppose. I feel about Truman rather the same as one does about an understudy. I'm sure he can go through the words and motions, but there is just not that spark of genius that makes the star. Poor understudy, I feel very sorry for him in a way. Roosevelt was such a great man and has been at the top for so long. Very hard indeed to follow.

What is this I hear about a very lushy piebald moustache? You know I hate you behind a moustache. See that it comes off before you land in England please.

It is wonderful not to *have* to have the blackout any more, but it is strange how many people put them up just the same. Habit is an odd master. I think it will take the British a long time to realise when they are finally no longer weighed under by rules and regulations of regimented warfare. If of course we *are* ever free again. Take care of yourself darling and get well, you'll be home soon.
All my love always, your M.

1. Rommel was one of the German leaders who could see that the war was lost. He was implicated in the attempt on Hitler's life in July 1944 and afterwards was offered a choice between trial and the more honourable option of suicide. He chose the latter on 4 October 1944.

Tam to Margaret — Germany, 25 April 1945

My Darling,

Since writing last we've moved again, still at a well-stocked farm, thank God. Your gritty letter arrived and I agree with everything you said. You've been wonderfully good, but I was worried about Mother's ankle and Gwynne being broke and it's a bloody feeling trying to keep in touch and having to ferret out where everybody is. The news is fantastic, and of course the war is over. It's ghastly to think that more of our people's lives should go on being lost because these insane people without control or communications or a hope in hell, nothing but the last hysterical screams on their radio, go on hoping for some last miracle, a new V weapon or some such fabulous nonsense.

Just heard the six o'clock news – Mussolini caught slinking over the Swiss frontier. I see there's an exhibition of pictures of the Camps,[1] go and see it.

A poor disjointed letter, but one's mind is in a busy whirl, first here, then there in a flurry. Not being English I get so excited, not like my phlegmatic brother officers.
Goodnight and my love to you always my Darling,
Tam

1. The Nazi concentration camps.

Margaret to Tam Two Gates, Sunday 29 April 1945

Beloved,

How the atrocity stories shocked, no shocked is not bad enough.[1] I've had that feeling in the pit of my stomach one has when you know something awful has happened on waking in the morning, before true consciousness has dawned. And something seems to keep urging me to do something about it. But what can I do but shudder and hate and remember and Tell. Your letter only made me feel the war horror more keenly. How can such a race breed bodies that appear normal and healthy? This I cannot understand. One would think that the bodies that perform such deeds would of God's will become degraded and wretched to behold. But no, the bestiality is only apparent in the eyes and expression. And even then not always. You've seen so much more than I darling, tell me why this should be? Human liver and heart, ye Gods! What a world to live in that a man and a woman who love each other and only desire to work and love and live in peace, should be actually writing these things to each other as truth never to be forgotten or forgiven. Oh darling if only they were all a bad dream and men who were tattooed were not murdered to make decorative lamp shades. I'm sick, I can't write, I loathe every rotten gutted son of a fucking bastard of them. But I adore you and always will my love, always, your M.

1. On 15 April the concentration camp at Belsen was liberated, followed two days later by Buchenwald.

Margaret to Tam Two Gates, Monday, (undated) 1945

Darling One,

I'm afraid I ended my last letter to you rather abruptly, but I do as you do too, get rather heated about the atrocities and I quite forgot to tell you lots of other little odds and ends.

Yes my darling the application has definitely gone in. So bless your heart get on with it, write to the Colonel and get back here as soon as possible. Oh and give me as much notice as you can darling, so that I can make some plans. Also I want to look my best, it takes a bit longer these days for me to tart myself up, you know!

Loo and Prue have been here all afternoon and are busy doing some fan mail for you and are furious at having to go back to school in case they miss the Victory. Any hour now, not a matter of days any more. It's amazing how quietly everyone is taking it, just a deep feeling of relief and gratitude to God and the men and women who have made it so.

Oh darling, how long do you think it will take them to let your application go through? It is too much to think you might be coming home any day now. I've got a dozen agents trying to find a house and if the worst comes to the worst we can carry on here for a few weeks, can't we my love?

Loo and Prue are going off now so I'll give them this to post. It is true, it is all coming true, you'll soon be home!!!!
God bless you and my love for always, Your M.

Tam to Margaret Germany, 30 April 1945

Darling,

So Johnny has been writing home about my moustache. It's quite black and not mottled and I'm keeping it this time for you to see for it's a beauty and it might make Hugo laugh.

The weekend has provided great excitement and rumours are flying thick and fast – Mussolini killed and Hitler dead – or is he? It will be the most appalling nuisance if the body is not produced, then for years there will be plots and counter plots and stories of his living in some mountain fortress preparing the Fourth Reich. Cerebral Haemorrhage the very day Berlin is assaulted sounds altogether too convenient. I can so well forsee the days to come when English tourists return from a spring in Bavaria with tales of a shepherd with a forelock and a silly moustache, or a café proprietor with a beard but with those unmistakable eyes! Napoleon was the most infernal nuisance during his captivity, and if Hitler is surrounded in any kind of mystery, if there's any doubt as to his death then we're in for a lot of expense and a lot of bother. The Peace proposals seem rather amateur, though the whole damn thing is so utterly disorganised now I doubt if a formal surrender would hasten the end of the actual fighting.

I see in the papers letters beginning to appear saying there are two Germanies, we must eradicate the Nazis but see that the rest of Germany is economically sound and productive. Germany must have her place in Europe – My God. If that idea is supported then the bloody six years of the world's agony has been utterly in vain. Thank God for the Russians, I believe they'll extract the ultimate penalties.

I can say 'Six eggs daily' very nicely now and then I shout

SCHNEL! very loud which I think means 'quickly'. Bastards I loathe them.

I have been trying for ten days to wangle my way into the camp at Belsen. Yesterday I went. I was a little nervous that I might be sick or have to leave, but the horrors were not the nauseating kind – the burials are now under some kind of control. The only dead one saw were those who had just collapsed – hideous and emaciated. I walked down one road and coming back a few minutes later there were two who had not been there before. No one paid attention to them. They might have been a couple of fish lying on the bank of a stream. The death rate is something like 400 a day still – starvation mostly, not Typhus – the birth rate about half a dozen. The filth was indescribable, and I did not venture inside the huts which must be far worse. The whole place was littered with old clothes and rags taken from the dead before burial, they were removed from the huts and burnt – they were smouldering still and here and there a flame where some ghastly creature was trying to use it to heat something. For quite some way – the roads were a foot high with these half-burnt rags – soaking from the rain and from the hosing. There was an enormous preponderance of women – which may have been that men were sent to the slave camps, but I believe that women are stronger than men and had survived in greater numbers. Of course there's a great many quite healthy plump girls and young women – these were the latest arrivals and somehow accentuated the horror of the starving. It was not quite like the Zoo and not quite like a Lunatic Asylum – but it had diabolical elements of both. I am quite certain I saw many, very many, who were mad. There was a dreadful sort of busy activity – women raking through a muddy rain-drenched heap of potato peelings – carefully and very methodically – and others fanning a flame amongst the rags – cooking their muck – or picking at garments from the debris which might give warmth or make a roof for an improvised tent. One felt unless they employed every waking moment to the business of survival they would have all been screaming. The desperate efforts were the only objective outlet they had – and so they continue until nature releases them from their misery. No that's wrong I think. I think for the most part that had already happened. When they went mad that was the end of their suffering. I wonder. I hope so. . . There was no attempt at any sort of privacy – latrines had no screening and people too tired or exhausted to reach them squatted where they were – oblivious and untroubled. I saw one old man – his legs bare, for some reason he was tearing up his pyjama trousers – and they were not as round as Hugo's.

He was quite mad I'm sure and his skin looked as if it didn't and never had fitted his bones. There were 60,000 in there last winter. It couldn't have been a secret kept by the SS or the Nazis from the rest of Germany. More, but not of this, later.
My love for always and always, Tam.

Later

Bernadotte gone again to Himmler.[1] Himmler, I take it, must have been dealt the worst hand. Goering packed up both figuratively and literally last week, Goebbels has not been heard of for days and Hitler reported dead. It looks very much as if Himmler had been left to fix a Peace while the others moved to new headquarters. It's all very like an objection, hanging about waiting anxiously, wondering when the 'alright flag' will go up, quite confident but terrified that something awful is taking place in the Stewards Room.
My love to Hugo, I'll see you both soon, I hope,
Tam

1. Count Folke Bernadotte (1895–1948), Swedish diplomat who conveyed Himmler's offer of capitulation to the British and US governments.

Margaret to Tam — Two Gates, 3 May 1945

My Darling,

I rang Sir David Cunningham from Con's myself and he told me that the application went in on April 16th definitely, and yesterday when I rang him he'd been on to the Board of Trade (who do these matters for them) to give them a reminder that they did need you urgently for a film to be started soon. I asked him what he thought the chances were and he said 50/50.

God the papers and news is so *fantastic* these days that one's inclined to refuse to take it all in. I have to go back sometimes and read the papers of yesterday and the day before to make sure I've not imagined these colossal and fantastic streaks of world history. Of course it is all over. I really thought the bells would ring on Tuesday sometime. *Hitler* dead, *Goebells*[*sic*] dead – suicides, I wonder. Or have they made a getaway, not being English!!! Oh dear and have you got a foreign accent now, you bloody little welch man with an English grandmother! You come home a tidy boy now and don't be getting into foreign ways look you!

God bless you my love and hurry home. All my love always and always, your M.

Tam to Margaret Germany, 6 May 1945

My Darling,

What a deal of excitement since my last letter and now it's all over and finished. I've no doubt that Victory in Europe Day will not be announced for some time but the great point is that the German Army is beaten. Absolutely and unarguably and completely beaten and it's a sweet sight to see them shambling down the roads in every kind of vehicle from armoured car to farmer's cart, bicycles and prams. Broken down motors being towed by trucks and lorries which look as though they'd fall apart at any moment. But sweeter still to see them straggling along on their flat feet and their rotten ersatz boots in the drizzling rain – abject, defeated, disillusioned and heavy with foreboding, with their countrymen watching them in every village and town, seeing the greatest army in the world reduced to a hungry, weary, disorganised shambles picking cigarette ends from the gutter where they'd been thrown by our troops. The Master Race hurrying into captivity, some of them with women and their wives and children in battered prams underneath a pile of cardboard suitcases, like the great stream of humanity to Epsom Downs on Derby Day, but instead of the holiday gaiety there's ultimate despair. No guards are necessary and they are herded into fields by the tens of thousands with no wire round them. There is only one solace to their shame and that is that they go to English camps and not Russian, for one and all are filled with terror of the Russians and from what one hears I'm happy to say with ample justification.

I heard a story today of an old German who inquired from an American Colonel who was occupying his home, if he intended to rape his daughter. When the American explained that we did not behave like that, the old man couldn't believe it or understand it. He knew the German Army raped and pillaged and he had been told that we should. It was inconceivable that we should not. Later when the American told him that very likely the Russians would ultimately occupy that area he fainted.

The roads, apart from being thronged with the surrendered German Armies, also have our own liberated prisoners-of-war – British, Canadian, Italian, Russian, American, Poles, and uniformed people who may be Hungarian. Then add in your imagination all the displaced families with all their goods and chattels, all the civilian refugees scuttling into western Germany out of the path of the dreaded Russians, and all in the drenching rain, on bad roads, constantly and continually having to jump in the ditch out of the way of traffic, trying to cross rivers in little boats when we close the bridges, hungry, homeless and frightened and wondering dumbly why they hadn't won the war, oh it's a great and glorious and unforgettable shambles.

I think possibly before I'd been to Belsen I might have had compassion for them, or at least a feeling of profound depression as I had when I saw what had been the city of Cologne, but now I find it immensely satisfactory and as I listen to the rain pattering on the tent I'm glad, for it is the one thing necessary to make their misery complete. For I know it is unutterable balls to pretend that the whole German race did not know of the existence of these camps and the horrors and agonies they contained. If people in England, now that the V weapons are finished, the Blitz now far away and the threat of invasion in 1940 just a rather amusing memory, would only realise they themselves escaped the same fate by a very narrow margin of good luck and great gallantry, we may see Germany really crushed and beyond resurrection. But enough of all of this. The war's won and we won it and now let's get on with our lives.

I had hoped that the end of the war would find me in some measure exhilarated, at least with the same sense of relief as you have when you walk out of the dentist or pay a pressing creditor, but no. Perhaps it will come when I leave the Army, that rather disgusting self-righteousness one feels over a duty discharged, but all I have at the moment is a cold fear that we shall bog it again. And with that fear I have another, a worse one. Before the war I thought that anyone who said the only good German is a dead one, was hateful, stupid, unimaginative, a fool, a blimp, a retired Army Clod – but now I believe it absolutely and I await the tragic moment when Hugo, hearing me say so, will think me all those things with ill-concealed scorn.

We've moved again and are likely to stay put – needless to say it's the worst camp site we've had.

See you soon I hope – I hope. God bless and all my love for always,
Tam

Tam to Margaret Germany, 8 May 1945 (VE Day)

Well My Beloved – the bloody thing is over at last and it is very fitting that I should be writing to you on the note paper of the Duke of Mecklenburg which I took from his palace the day before yesterday. The BBC last night climbed to new heights of hitherto undiscovered bathos – after telling us the historic news we've all been waiting and working for for so many years they finished with these words: 'Cotton Bunting may be purchased without coupons until the end of May'. And so today and all its anniversaries I shall call Bunting Day.

Yesterday I went to another concentration camp at Ludwigslust. I saw a party of fifty civilians being conducted through the horrors, a mixed party of both men and women. Only three of the women showed any signs of emotion, the rest showed nothing but sullen ill temper. These same civilians in the morning had dug two hundred graves immediately in front of Mecklenburg's Palace.

The whole town was made to file past the bodies before burial and remain for the service. I talked to a cameraman, an American who was filming the conducted party. He told me he's had instructions from London to lay off the horror stuff, the editors couldn't take it.

And here is the best story of the war, Field Marshal Milch surrendered to Mills-Roberts who commands the 1st Commando Brigade – he arrived in tremendous state complete with baton – during the conversation Mills-Roberts said to him, 'You were here in this area, you must have known about these camps.' 'Certainly,' said Milch. 'Well why didn't you do something about them?' 'But they were not people like us, you or I – they were Poles and Russians mostly – muck – not like us.' Whereupon Mills-Roberts saw very red and seizing the Field Marshal's baton broke it over his head. Milch was taken off for medical attention and Mills-Roberts has the two broken pieces of the baton as about the best souvenir a man ever had. I think it's magnificent and the Poet Laureate should make a ballad of it.

What the hell we do now God knows. As long as I can get out and about and see the country and the filthy swine either caged or hobbling down the roads I shan't be bored. I wonder what you'll be up to tonight? I should dearly like to see the King on the balcony of his Palace – a Great Day.

Soon now my darling Margaret – and we must make up to each other for all the wretchedness and loneliness of these hateful years.

From now on anyway the suffering of Europe will decrease so that that part of one's conscience can be a little easier and we can be happy without feeling guilty, only terribly, terribly, unbelievably lucky.
I shall love you always my darling,
Tam

.

Tam to Margaret Germany, 13 May 1945

My darling,

I've just been reading Friday's papers giving details and forecast of demobilisation. Those parts of it I understood seemed profoundly depressing and I gathered no Class B people will be dealt with yet and my A Class won't get out until September. It's now a month since the application went in and I must know if it's yes or no. I know you've done everything you can but get on to Connie. I cannot and will not have this ghastly period of ill-temper and impatience and strained nerves and boredom with nothing to do for a third time. Not that things are bloody yet, but I can see the symptoms.

I had another very interesting day on Friday, went up to Kiel. On the way we stopped at a farm and made them boil us some eggs. A very good looking, very blonde fellow came and saluted. He was a Polish Officer captured in '39 and had spent five years in the concentration camp at Auschwitz in Poland. He worked in one of the five crematoria, each capable of 5000 bodies a day. All the usual frightful stories, eleven million he reckoned while he was working there. Now he prefers working on a farm for Germans than being re-patriated to Russian-occupied Poland. What a hideous problem it all is, God knows how it will all end and sort out. He was a charmer. Kiel was flat as a pancake, and it did one good to see the entire population, every single person, nobody was doing anything else, old, young, man, woman and child clearing the rubble and the dusty ruins away in shopping bags and slop pails, buckets, suitcases, anything which would carry debris. Their hearts must have been filled with gall, nothing in the world is more infuriating than clearing up somebody else's mess and it'll take them months. Passed thousands and thousands of tramping Bosche returning from Denmark, tired, dusty, hot, sweating – some SS Bastards too. We went right over all the Dock area and climbed aboard the Hippe[1] – bombed to buggery – and saw the U-Boat

pens and one and two men submarines. They must have been brave men. Horribly unsafe and lonely looking things.
No more now Beloved. Longing to hear from you about V.E. celebrations. My love always, always,
Tam

1. The *Admiral von Hippe* was a cruiser.

Margaret to Tam Two Gates, 15 May 1945

Beloved,

Oh my darling I really think this is the worst period of the war, at any rate the worst for a long time. The fighting is all over in Europe and being apart seems so senseless now – more than ever a waste of time. Everyone seems to be busily getting their lives into order or being madly gay and all I want to do at the moment is to find a house and get ready for you to come back to us. You too must be feeling madly restless and bored for there can surely be no job for you at all now. Charles says there are about ninety thousand officers in England now with no jobs (returned P.O.W.s included) who have to wait about for their demob time to come round. It does seem ridiculous, doesn't it?

Everyone who I've met recently who has just returned is filled with the same loathing and determination not to be soft this time. For this alone I'm glad. I could not have born to have heard that the 'Hun is quite human after all' from any man's lips. I wonder now sometimes how ever we got through the years of the war – so often apart when we needed each other most. But I shall always be grateful that you were with me for Hugo and those happy days just before and after. Even now looking back I realise how terribly important it is for a man and a woman to be together at such a time. You were right we must be together – it would have been a miserable time to have had Hedda while you were away. I suppose that is why we did not start another. We are meant to be together when babies are coming. Do you agree darling?

Mummy and I are clearing the house out and getting rid of all the odds and ends we've kept during the war 'just in case', which clutter this tiny house up so much. We are also sleeping and eating just when we please, and clearing ourselves out after Victory week.

Your Victory letter was very neat and orderly. I quite expected an alcoholic scrawl darling. Yes Bunting Day is an excellent name. The B.B.C. never fails, do they? The Mills Roberts story is terrific. Certainly a great poem should be written about it. How wonderful.

I'll run now darling and try and catch the four o'clock post. God bless you and see you soon now thank the Lord. Always I'll love you,
Your own Margaret.

Margaret to Tam Two Gates, 18 May 1945

My darling,

Still no news your end or this end about the application. The buggers who deal with such things have lost it in their celebrations I'll bet. But darling I'm sure it will come through by the end of this month. I'm so certain in my heart that I'll see you by the end of the month that *it must be so*. You are quite right, what on earth is the sense of waiting about being bored to death when there are jobs for you to go to. I don't see why the whole of Phantom aren't back anyway.

That Pole you met must have had a horrible time, what a miserable position to find oneself in, working for the Hun rather than return to one's own. Oh God, how will it all end for the people of the other European countries? Up at 5.30 yesterday and off to Welwyn[1] for my test. Never been so nervous in all my life. I just shook and shook and shook. In fact I did a very bad test. So I think I'm out darling and will be able to join you with E.N.S.A. *Are you mad*, do you think I'm going to let you go to Burma without me? Even for E.N.S.A. I won't let you go away again. Oh please don't darling, I want you here so badly. Do come home soon, I implore you, please!

Must fly now darling, going to catch the bus to Windsor for some shopping.

I love you my beloved and I want you home badly – no, I want *you* badly.
Always and always
Your own M.

1. Film studios at Welwyn Garden City.

Tam to Margaret Germany, 23 May 1945

My Darling,

These bloody mails have gone to hell. Only two letters from you since May 6th. I know from past experience that these letters one is waiting for now will simply never turn up – the modern method of censorship is simply to withhold altogether.

Been away for a couple of days to Holland to pick up a radiator for one of my vehicles. The roads were fearful and I feel as though I've ridden there and back on a camel.

It was a relief to get out of Germany, the atmosphere is odious, like sharing a dressing room with a man with whom you're not on speaking terms. The bastards are so damn obliging and civil that in spite of the fact that all one's instincts are to kick their teeth in, it's a continual effort to be frigid and short and sharp in your dealings with them. When a man takes endless trouble to cut your hair it's hard not to say 'Thank you, that's very good', and when children wave it's only natural to wave back, but one doesn't of course and as I say the atmosphere is bloody, so that it was heaven to smile and say hallo and give people cigarettes again.

The sex side of non-fraternisation is of course an enormous problem and no effort is being made to cope with it. The Russians, if they don't actually encourage rape, certainly countenance it, and the French of course establish brothels. But England in her usual idiotic way refuses to recognise the existence of sex and a man is court-martialled if he even smiles at a girl. The girls have got turned on to this and swish about in their summer frocks. I saw some sun bathing near Hamburg the other day in only shorts. To men who've endured a year's bloody fighting and a cold winter suddenly to feel warm again and to be relieved of continual danger and discomfort and horror, it's sheer lunacy to imagine that the one thing filling their minds and bodies isn't the dire necessity for a thumping good bang. The Army's solution is P.T. and Games. Dear God give me patience with the English, for they are strange and not as other men.

I sent my Patrol into town to the pictures – they stood in a queue for an hour and then didn't get in. I suppose all the bloody Actors are so busy making their little pile of gold – damn their miserable, well-cut souls. I really and honestly and truly will have to be watched very carefully when I get back – it'll take me a long time to forget how unspeakably most of them – some of them – have behaved. This isn't an oblique way of saying 'I've done damn well, I have', nothing could be wronger, my war's been lucky, interesting and fairly steady. It's just that I think they're a lot of large, prosperous and quite horrible rats. I shall avoid the larger of their holes like the Ivy and the Grill[1] for the sight of them munching with their sharp little rodent teeth revolts me.

God bless you my Pretty Margaret and give Hugo my love. I've got to the pitch now when I cannot think of him or you or the girls or make plans or look forward any more – it's too near and delay now is awful. I love you – I always shall. Always.
Tam

1. The Ivy and the Savoy Grill, both popular restaurants with actors.

Tam to Margaret Germany, 26 May 1945

My Darling,

Tremendous excitement here a couple of days ago over Himmler's suicide, and a certain amount of concern, for they reckoned on getting a lot out of him about the German underground organisation. Someone came round and asked if I'd like to see his body – not a thing I really wanted to do just before tea, however I went along.[1] I've seen so many dead people in various states and with widely varying emotions – I've been horrified and awed and saddened and nauseated. The dead I've seen have mostly been grotesque for I don't think I've seen anyone who died a natural or peaceful death – but looking at Himmler – not a pleasant sight when alive I should imagine – excited nothing in me except delight and joy. Not only the war seemed more over and finished than before, but all the agony and butchery and torture. The cameras were clicking nineteen to the dozen and every part of his horrible body was photographed from every angle – this not for the press but for identification. An insignificant face, nothing vile or cruel about it, he might have been a clerk or a waiter. Give a little man who should be adding up a cash book the most powerful position in Europe, second only to a house painter, and it's a logical progression and quite inevitable that you find the pit at Belsen. I hear good reports from there by the way. It's extraordinary that the least horrible thing I remember of Belsen was the gallows. I see the Archbishop of Canterbury has a letter in the *Telegraph* saying 'In spite of the evidence of these terrible camps we must not blind ourselves to the fact that there are good Germans'. I should like to tell him that Pontius Pilate was good to his mother and Iscariot was fond of cats! Dear Holy God it puts murder in one's heart, what are we to do, what are we to do? Or am I wrong? Perhaps I'm terribly wrong, unchristian and inhuman. I don't know. But I know if I'd had a tendency to blood pressure I should have burst before now.

How is Hugo? My love and a kiss on the back of his neck to him. Don't let him think it's my fault I'm still here.

God bless you my darling, I adore you, write to me. Always and forever,

Tam

1. By this time Tam had arrived in Berlin.

Margaret to Tam — Two Gates, Whitsun 1945

Tamèd beloved,

Unfortunately I've been unable to badger Connie since your letter arrived yesterday morning on account of it is Whit. Also I gather that they are turning down nearly all applications and the best way and almost the only way now is through E.N.S.A., so I'll have to change my mind for I'd give anything to get you out soon darling. I'm also told that all applications are taking between 6 and 7 weeks to be looked at and either OK'd or turned down. It's just five weeks now so I'd give them a bit longer and allow for the peace hols too.

I should hear just how bad my test was during the week. Oh God darling I was awful. Maybe it's just as well, now I shall probably be free to join you with E.N.S.A. if they'll have us together. How would you like to go to Italy? I would, much more than the Far East.

It's a bloody day, cold and rainy.

All my love, always and always,

Your own M.

Margaret to Tam — Two Gates, Wednesday, 30 May 1945

My beloved,

Still no definite news in spite of repeated requests to Connie. She says to tell you that they really are keeping at it and that as soon as there is any news she'll ring me at once. As I told you in a previous letter darling, they finally did not ask for you until mid-June, thinking you'd have a better chance of coming out with the first demob on or about June 18th. And now Connie tells me they won't start work on *Lottie Dundas* until July – I suppose Vivien's play in London has been a success and may run. Oh dear, you still seem keen to do this E.N.S.A. trick, after so long darling. Six years in the army very nearly, I can't bear to think of you going away again once I get you home. Well damn and FUCK. I've been so sure for so long that the next time would be for good and no more goodbyes. Just a steady run together darling. Oh the bloody thing *must* come through.

Wonder how you got on with the Col – perhaps by now you've settled it and are coming home. Or perhaps – God I hope so – you are all being sent back to Richmond.[1]

You will have had my letter telling you about the house I saw on Monday by the time you get this. It really is not at all bad, as I told you, furniture not fantastic, but roomy and high up and a lovely garden. I forgot to tell you that there is a 9 hole golf course just beyond the woods of the garden and it is 39 miles from London and 22 from Windsor. There is a lovely view as it is 500′ up and central heating in the main rooms, as well as gas fires. Two permanent gardeners who are included in the 12 guineas a week rent. I've told you a lot of this before darling but I thought I'd better as you don't seem to be getting all my letters Tam. I don't think I've had all of yours either darling. I've *never* written you less than four a week and sometimes more so the mails must have gone *nuts*.

Still no news of my test. I'm told they expect to decide the cast by next weekend. Oh God, this waiting for other people to make up their minds about us is making me ill with suspense and I imagine you are in the same state my love.

Oh time, time, hurry by and bring good news quickly.
Goodnight my most precious darling,
Always and always, your M.

1. Phantom's English headquarters.

Tam to Margaret — Germany, 16 June 1945

My Darling,

This is timed to reach you on the 21st so as to bring you my love upon that most important day, but I daresay the bloody mails will fail me. This is the third wedding anniversary we've been away from each other, my beloved, and by God it shall be the last. We must never forget these years of difficulty when we're happy, otherwise we may get lazy with our happiness, take it for granted and end up by forgetting that it's there. I wish so enormously I could be with you, to take you somewhere exquisite for dinner, with special flowers and food and a little padded box in my pocket burning its way through my dinner jacket until exactly the right moment to produce it, meanwhile a magnum cooling itself in a pretty bedroom and gardenias waiting on your shoulder for their merciless destruction. I should then be able to make you really know how the years have made me love you more than I did on that beautiful blue day in 1940. And how I thank you for making me happy, and for making the worries so worth while, and for all the comfort and the fun and the joy of being your lover and the happiness of being your husband – which two delicious occupations I shall be at again now my love, within measurable distance – eight weeks in all, maybe sooner. The looking forward to it is unbearable and I try not to imagine it. A little later when it's nearer maybe.

My love to Hugo and ask him to kiss your hands for me, soon now my most beloved, soon. I go on loving you so much and I always shall,
Tam

Tam to Margaret — Germany, 24 June 1945

My Darling,

I have written to you at length telling you to contact Peter Chappell at the Mess at Richmond who has some stuff of mine which you will please collect. I hope he manages to get it back and that you can pick it up, on account of the house we have the Mess in burnt down the night before last and it represents all I have left. I was playing backgammon in my shirt and corduroys when the panic started at about 6.30. My room was unfortunately on the top floor and by 7.30 all I possessed was my shirt and corduroys. I looked in vain later but nothing was even distinguishable. Two little blue stones for you, some pictures and all sorts of odds and ends that I had collected for you as well as everything of mine – papers, notebooks, cigars, every stitch of clothing, boots, shoes, the whole lot.[1] I went up to have a look but it wasn't on to try to get them. Things aren't worth getting upset about and certainly not worth getting burnt for. I now have a vile new battle dress and a beret with no badge, two shirts and issue shaving stuff, so I shall leave the Army as I entered it, with the private soldier's minimum.

I can hardly believe that in eight weeks I shall be with you in England and out of this infected horrible country, and shot of the

Army for ever and ever. It's really quite miserable here. No work, and this frightfully depressing atmosphere of no fraternisation. Terrible scenes during the fire. I thought one girl was going to hit me, and then two very amateur German firemen got badly hurt when a bit of the house fell on them. I felt they thought we'd done it on purpose, which I hated.
My love always and always,
Tam

1. Tam must have kept Margaret's letters separate from the rest of his kit because these were not destroyed in the fire.

Margaret to Tam Two Gates, Monday, (undated) June 1945

Now my beloved,

At last I can make some definite plans for your return, because until your letter arrived today I was in a bit of a quandry [*sic*] about booking rooms etc. It is even more difficult to get rooms now I believe, and I imagine you'd rather spend the first night or two at Claridges or somwhere like that where we can get drunk and anything else we may need. Oh God I'm excited darling. I've been home and collected your stuff and I was able to goose your bootmakers, shirtmakers and tailor into being ready for you. BASTARDS ALL!!!

The latest from Connie is that Tony de Grunwald (can't spell it) has written a play and wants you for it. He says it is a lovely part and that Terrence [*sic*] Rattigan is putting money into it. Binkie[1] is producing too I gather darling.

I want you to get this as soon as possible my love so that you know my plans for you. I'm longing for the day my beloved and terribly excited. I adore you always and always, your M.

1. Binkie was the nickname of Hugh Beaumont, one of the most prolific theatre producers of the time.

Tam to Margaret Germany, 30 June 1945

My Darling,

I went down to Belsen a couple of days ago. It was just about nine weeks since I was there. Still 1700 at Belsen, 7000 in hospital. The work done by the doctors and medical students and nursing staff has been tremendous. A little Red Cross welfare girl – 22 years old – showed me No.4 Camp where most of the healthy women internees are now quartered. It's the only thing I've seen in Germany where intelligence and vision and humanity have been employed. Five Red Cross girls have done it all and must have worked like slaves. But oh how splendid to see them with a real light of purpose in their eyes! They've restored the self respect of these people so brilliantly – little competitions for the best rooms and the prettiest flowers – sewing rooms, games rooms, music rooms, studio, reading and writing and news rooms, a theatre going – concerts and dances. These girls had all arrived on April 19th, three days after it was uncovered, and had nursed and buried the sick and dead in all that unspeakable stench and horror. My God they made me nearly cry with admiration. I asked this funny little mousey girl with buck teeth and a shy manner and the amazing name of Miss Gotobed what they now needed most – 3000 toothbrushes and toothpaste she said, and one wanted to rush all over Europe getting them for her.

My love to you always my darling,

Tam

Margaret to Tam — Two Gates, 4 July 1945

My darling,

Letter from you this morning. Miss Gotobed and her companions must be wonderful people, how proud they must be to have done such a grand job of work. And how interesting for you to have seen it before and after as it were! Even now when I think of the horror of the stories I read and heard about those camps I feel sick and full of hate and loathing. I talked to an Australian the other day, he had been a P.O.W. for four years. He seemed convinced that there will be yet another war more horrible than this in ten to fifteen years. Oh God darling, surely civilisation can not be mad and blind enough to let it happen again. It would be the end of the world I'm sure. Science will by then be so colossally developed that even our wildest imaginations could not fathom its possibilities. No one could survive.

Four to six weeks! Oh my darling it is almost too good to be true. It's about the first plan you've been able to write to me in six years that we were certain of being carried out. Always the army was in the background with an invisible hand ready to say do this do that, go here go there. And at last we know that in six weeks at the outside it will be done with forever. Hooray hooray my love.

We are going to a furniture sale after lunch. Everything bloody expensive, but not bad down here. A lot of stuff from bombed out houses I think.

Hugo was saying Gentle Jesus to me last night when I heard him say very earnestly 'Suffer me to come to tea'. Oh dear what a foolish muddle prayers must seem to him at his age.

God bless you my beloved, see you soon soon soon. All my love darling now and always and always,
Your M.

Margaret to Tam — Two Gates, 20 July 1945

Beloved,

Just a short note to enclose the latest letter from the agents about White Leaf House[1]. Denham is nearer than I thought and Amersham further, so you can see how good I am at map reading darling.

A beastly windy rainy day today so I suppose that it is indoor sport for poor old Hugo. How he loves the sun too.

Only nine more days my love and then our life begins together. I just hope and pray everything will go well for you my love and that I can in some measure make up to you for the bloody years of sacrifice you've made. I hope I can make you laugh and be happy for always. It seems so strange that we have been married for five years, together for nearly eight years, and yet we've never really had a home together where we could plan ahead and rule our own lives as we wished. I wonder how and where we'd be now if there'd been no war.

God bless you my love and I'll be seeing you in nine days!!!!
Always and always,
Your own M.

1. Tam and Margaret moved in to White Leaf House near Princes Risborough when he returned to England.

Tam to Margaret — 23 July 1945

I leave here on the 30th. I look forward to the process with great misgivings and anticipate delay and Bog. I am prepared to find myself in Sunderland or South Wales waiting for inoculation – or a Court of Inquiry into the loss of my compass by fire – or a copy of my decree Nisi – there will be storms at sea – fog in the Channel

– a case of Enteric Fever on the ship and quarantine at Southend for three weeks – anything may happen from mistaken identity to loss of memory – so expect me when you see me. If after two months there is no sign of me begin telephoning influential people. At present I am searching for the Army File Unit. My military Identity Card was burnt and I can find no-one to photograph me for my new one. This may cause months of delay. The Air Photography Intelligence Section can only snap me from 20,000 feet, the Field Security Police have courteously offered, in the event of my not being photographed, to take my finger prints. I hear *One of Our Aircraft is Missing* is on in Copenhagen and am wondering if I might get hold of a couple of reels of that – but the R.A.F. uniform would confuse everybody and might have *terrifying* results. Another peculiar thing, I entered the Territorial Army without a medical examination – I was embodied into the Regular Army without one – I survived six years without one – but now, within a few days of my release, I've had the most extensive going over of my whole life, the whole works. At the end of which I was marked 'Fit for further Service' which rather depressed me.

Thank you my darling for all the letters through all these years – one would have thought your writing and spelling would have improved with practice, but no. Though your text, I must admit, is fuller and more robust than the evening when all you wrote was TAM TAM TAM TAM TAM – but there was something in it that made my heart leap like a salmon in a pool. Till I see you next and then for always,
Tam

Postscript

Tam's fears about losing his place in the theatre proved to be well-founded. In the post-war years he had to struggle to re-establish himself professionally. Between 1945 and 1950 he was in *Zoo in Silesia*, a play about a prisoner-of-war camp, at the Embassy Theatre in Swiss Cottage, and of the half dozen films in which he appeared, only Oscar Wilde's *An Ideal Husband* was of any note. During this time he tried to give Margaret, Hugo and their new baby Simon the wonderful life that they had all been dreaming of, with the result that in the early 1950s expenditure was way outstripping income, and he was declared a bankrupt.

Devastating though this must have been for all the family, in some ways it proved a blessing. Tam was forced to use every resource available and as work was still scarce, the idea occurred to him that he should try and write a play with a starring part for himself. In 1956 he opened in *Plaintiff in a Pretty Hat* which he wrote with Margaret's help. It proved to be a smash hit. Eight other plays followed, including the musical *Charlie Girl* which ran for six years, a record only broken by Andrew Lloyd Webber. At one time three of his plays were on in the West End and two of them, *The Grass is Greener* and *Flip Side*, were made into films. Using his wits and his considerable talents Tam was able to redeem himself.

Simon's birth in 1946 was followed by the arrival of a daughter, Polly, in 1950. Like many show-business marriages, Tam and Margaret's ebbed and flowed. Nonetheless they proved a successful writing team and this, coupled with the bonds forged between them during the war, helped their marriage to survive until Tam's death at the age of sixty-five in December 1969, three days after he had opened in the West End in *His Hers and Theirs*, yet another of their own plays. In it he and Margaret had written a part for their son Simon as well. Margaret outlived Tam by twenty-five years, filling his role as head of the family. They are both still affectionately remembered and this book is a loving tribute to them.

Index